PRAISE FOR *THE*

"The shaming we go through as women is incredible. We even shame each other. It's about time someone called it out and gave us the tools to reclaim our everyday joy and honest expression. *The Goddess Guides* are a **world changer**. Well done, Ava."
—International Bestseller Kate Perry aka Kathia Zolfaghari, Artist & Activist

"Emboldened, shocking and necessary, *The Goddess Guides to Being a Woman* is a **life-changing journey** every woman will want to take."
—Crystal Andrus Morissette, Founder of the S.W.A.T. Institute (Simply Woman Accredited Trainer)

"Author Ava Miles redefines and alters the experience of shame for women and for the men who love them. Power comes from the way you speak and listen. Miles' series is an **exquisite exploration** of internal discomfort and courage, allowing you to reclaim your divine soul and fully express your womanhood. I highly recommend."
—Dr. Shawne Duperon, Project Forgive Founder, Nobel Peace Prize Nominee

"After being raped in college, I believe that all work for the empowerment of women is important, essential. This Goddess series creates a movement towards this effort of **awakening women to their power** – power which is limitless, in truth. Ava Miles is a courageous fellow writer whose mission is to empower all women."
—Aspen Matis, author of the internationally bestselling memoir, *Girl in the Woods*

"Ava **gets to the heart** of why some of us do toxic or hang around drama while helping us all realize we can have happy and loving relationships that don›t clutter up our space or make us sick."
—Courtney Cachet, Celebrity Designer & TV Personality

ALSO BY AVA MILES

The Calendar of New Beginnings
Home Sweet Love
The Moonlight Serenade
Daring Brides

The Dare River Series

Country Heaven
Country Heaven Song Book
Country Heaven Cookbook
The Chocolate Garden
The Chocolate Garden:
A Magical Tale (Children's Book)
Fireflies and Magnolias
The Promise of Rainbows
The Fountain of Infinite Wishes

Dare Valley Meets Paris Billionaire Mini-Series

The Billionaire's Gamble
The Billionaire's Courtship
The Billionaire's Secret
The Billionaire's Return

To Helen —

goddesses
eat

Reclaiming a Divine
Partnership with Food

*Here's to being
an amazing
goddess woman ...*

Ava Miles

Ava Miles

Legal Disclaimer

This book is solely for entertainment purposes. The author and publisher are not offering it as professional services and it is not intended to give medical, legal, accounting, or other professional services advice. While best efforts have been used in preparing this book, the author and publisher make no representations or warranties of any kind and assume no liabilities of any kind with respect to the accuracy or completeness of the contents and specifically disclaim any implied warranties of merchantability or fitness of use for a particular purpose. Neither the author nor the publisher shall be held liable or responsible to any person or entity with respect to any loss or incidental or consequential damages caused, or alleged to have been caused, directly or indirectly, by the information or programs contained herein. No warranty may be created or extended by sales representatives or written sales materials. Every person and/or company is different and the advice and strategies contained herein may not be suitable for your situation. You should seek the services of a competent professional before beginning any health or improvement program.

Although the examples in this book may reflect real-life situations, they aren't necessarily descriptions of actual people but in some cases are composites created from the author's views and personal experience. The story and its characters and entities are fictional. Any likeness to actual persons, either living or dead, is strictly coincidental, unless otherwise stated.

ISBN-10: 1-940565-78-2
ISBN-13: 978-1-940565-78-1
www.avamiles.com
Ava Miles

This one's going out to my grandmother, Lanone Miles, for both showing me and teaching me the love and joy of cooking and eating and how recipes connect us across the ages to loved ones past.

TABLE OF CONTENTS

The Goddess Guides

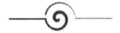

Introduction

We're all goddesses and gods in a body.

The first time I heard this declaration, I knew on a soul level it was true. In my Catholic upbringing, I commonly heard I was a child of God. When I grew up, I wasn't a child anymore, but instead of being accepted as a goddess in a body, I was told I was human, and as such, imperfect.

The human part is right. The imperfect part is not.

If you're reading this, you've come awake to the truth like me. You've remembered you're a goddess or god in a body.

My goddess nature—my higher self or my soul—is the perfect one. She helps me remember my true nature, the one that is simply love and joy. As such, my goddess side is dealing with the choice to incarnate and learning to live in this sometimes perfect, sometimes imperfect world where there are all these constructs. One of the most powerful ones is gender.

What does it mean to be a woman, especially a woman on your own terms?

And when you remember you're really a goddess in a body, what does it mean to be a woman *then*?

I like to use the term goddess woman here. My experience is that once you realize you are a goddess woman, *everything* changes. You relate differently to yourself, your relationships, and the world around you.

Why? Because when you open yourself to experiencing divine love and joy in a body, it invariably translates into being a new woman somehow.

A goddess woman.

And you aren't the only one who will experience a changed perspective. Those who know and love you and those you encounter will relate to you differently too.

These guides are meant to share what my goddess nature has taught me and is still teaching me about being a woman. I've had many spiritual awakenings, but seeing myself as a goddess woman was one of the most powerful shifts I've ever experienced.

It happened when I was meditating on a full moon—no joke—and suddenly I saw myself lying naked on a lily pad on the water. That woman was beautiful, and I realized for the first time in my life that *I* was beautiful. Me! The girl who had always thought she was just okay looking but made up for it by being super smart and hard-working. I finally saw the woman some people had called "pretty."

She wasn't just pretty, though. She was beautiful and wise, sexy and confident, lying there naked.

Before that day, I had a lot of shame around my body, about not being skinny enough, not looking like whoever the most popular model or actress was at the time.

I also didn't have confidence in myself as a woman, one who knew she was perfect and loveable—just as she was.

From then on, whenever I looked in the mirror, I looked for *her*. Me, the Goddess Woman. I didn't find her everyday. Sometimes I was too distracted by a bad hair day or extra weight after the holidays. Sometimes I got caught up in doubts about myself or my decisions. But I never stopped looking for her. And you know what? The more I looked, the more I saw her.

Seeing her—that gorgeous goddess woman—gave me the courage to do things I never would have done. Including quitting a very successful career rebuilding warzones to launch myself as a published author. Including writing these guides, the topics of which rather astounded my woman-self. But my goddess nature knew what was best for me.

So does yours.

There is no order to reading the series of books that make up *The Goddess Guides to Being a Woman*. You will read them in the order your soul intends. Some guides may resonate more than others.

Each guide highlights a different divine formula. These formulas are recipes for love, happiness, and wholeness from our goddess woman selves that have gotten buried under a slew of personal experience, confusion about our true nature, and the insidious specter shame wreaks on our lives, on our very selves. Together, they form a path that will lead us to the fullest expression of our goddess woman selves.

We're also going to hear stories about goddess women and their journeys. We've been learning how to be goddess women for centuries through storytelling, much of it oral until recent times. The modern myths contained in these guides are composites of women everywhere, some of whom I've met, some of whom I've heard about. These stories are intended to demonstrate core lessons and elucidate wisdom to help all of us goddess women navigate our way through life.

But there is a flip side to stories—while they can provide guidance and share wisdom, so too can they keep us locked in unloving and unhappy patterns. The stories we tell ourselves again and again (even if they're not true), and the stories we take on from others, making them our own, can lead to a life and self very disconnected from our goddess nature. So we're going to spend some intentional time examining the stories we each carry (and the beliefs embedded in them) and identify the ones that are keeping us from feeling like we're goddesses in a body. Then we're going to delete them through what I call "Reclaiming Practices." As a goddess woman with spiritual healing gifts, I've learned this is one of the fastest and most effective ways to reconnect with and embody our goddess woman selves. By setting this unwanted baggage down, we can begin to experience love and joy as our normal course of being and live the highest version of our lives. We're also going to talk about a variety of goddess woman tools proven to support our goddess woman nature and journey.

Ultimately, your soul knows what you need if you're not certain. All you have to do is be willing to engage in this journey honestly and with as much love for yourself as you can muster. That's where the magic and miracles are, and they're waiting for you if you want them.

You need only ask.

No spiritual teacher worth his or her salt should ever profess to have all the truths of the Universe. I certainly don't. But I was called to write these guides, and I had help from above. One thing I've known since I started writing my first book many books ago is that I wasn't writing alone. When I surrendered to that truth, miraculous things happened. I changed. More readers found me. I hit the bestseller charts time and time again.

When you're a goddess woman living in alignment with her soul purpose, the whole Universe rises to support you, like you've heard before. The right people find you. You found me, and on a soul-level, I found you.

Listen to your intuition. It can never lead you wrong.

Since I'm a goddess learning how to be a woman—a goddess woman—the highest version of being a woman, not the crap I was taught or forced to believe—these guides are geared toward that experience. And for all the lesbians reading this, I encourage you to substitute female pronouns and the like wherever it's appropriate. My wording isn't meant to be exclusive. I'm only speaking from my experience as a heterosexual goddess woman.

Some of these truths will also resonate for men. We're all humans, after all. Again, while these guides are not meant to be exclusive, I'm going to confine myself to talking about goddesses and women, not gods and men. Those guides are meant to be written by a man who is called to share his truth. I wish him and the men in the world well. They need to remember who they are too.

In the meantime, though, it's going to be just us goddess women.

Happy reading and great spiritual shifting.

Much love and light,

Ava

CHAPTER 1

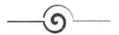

RECLAIMING OUR DIVINE FORMULA: GODDESS+FOOD=NOURISHMENT

How have so many of us gotten epically messed up about food?

There's no getting around it. We *have* to eat. Food is the fuel for our goddess bodies. That's not just a fact of life; it's a divine formula:

Goddess+Food=Nourishment

Nourishment is what helps our bodies grow and be healthy, but it has the potential to be more than that. This is where the Latin origin of the word gives us a helpful nudge: nourishment means to feed *and* cherish. That's right. When we eat as goddess women, we're also feeding our souls—

eating is an act of cherishing who we are. If you haven't had much cherishing in your life, it's the sweet, loving affection you have for yourself, something we're bringing back as part of our goddess transformation.

Why wouldn't we want this to be one of our divine truths? And yet, when we look at the relationship women have with food these days, many of us have gotten out of whack with this simple formula. Big time. As we discussed in *Goddesses are Sexy*, staying thin and looking like X super model or actress has become an obsession in Western society. In pursuit of this ideal, many women choose to go from diet to diet, keeping up with the latest craze. We have a whole subculture of women who subsist only on salads.

Many of us aren't enjoying food anymore, and if we do, we often feel guilty about it later.

Some women are so stringent in the "food is bad" mentality, they shame the people around them for eating, even going so far as to limit their daughters' food intake or insist they diet to live up to this super-thin "ideal" of womanhood.

Is it any wonder a staggering number of women around the world have eating disorders? Women are starving their goddess bodies, compulsively eating, or inducing violent vomiting after teasing our bodies with the nourishment it needs to be healthy. Maybe your own struggle with food has brought you to this guide.

Then there's the flip side of our issues with food.

What are we to make of the soaring obesity rates? The World Health Organization (WHO) Obesity and Overweight Fact Sheet from 2016 says there are close to two billion adults over eighteen years of age who are overweight. Six hundred million of those are obese; this is out of a world population of around eight billion. That's almost eight percent, folks.

Still with me? I know these numbers are staggering. Let's all take a deep breath and keep reading. According the American Health Association, in the United States (my home country) one in three adults is obese. Think of it. Out of every three people you or I meet, one of them is going to be obese.

Our children are becoming obese at earlier ages as well, and this is even true of cultures where obesity is historically uncommon according to the WHO—including non-sub-Saharan countries in Africa, I was shocked to learn (I used to work there in my old career). The statistics for obesity in these places, largely urban areas, have more than doubled in the past thirty years.

Diabetes has become an epidemic around the world, with the highest incidence in the United States, India, and China. But heart issues and other health problems related to over-consumption are also becoming a factor—as well as all the pills people are taking to tackle these problems.

How do women fit into the mix? Some of us handle stress and emotion through binge eating, which may lead to wild swings in our weight. Our personal stories can turn the foods we like most into "treats"—rewards for good behavior—or vices we hate ourselves for indulging in. This relationship often trickles down to our children: many parents use food as a carrot or a stick: "Sweetie, if you go potty, Mommy will give you a snack," or "You won't get dessert if you don't finish your vegetables."

But our problems with food aren't just linked to body weight, are they?

People appear to be suffering from food allergies at a higher level than ever recorded. We see gluten-free and dairy-free products overtaking natural products like bread and milk, staples to our ancestors.

Then we've got what I'll call system-level issues about food. And they run the gamut...

Scientists, the medical community, and the food industry are *constantly* telling us what's healthy or not healthy for us to consume—and the information is often confusing, conflicting, and changeable.

Organic produce is now considered better than conventional produce. A whole bunch of fruits, vegetables, and nuts have suddenly become "super foods." Grilling used to be bad for you due to carcinogens, but that fear craze seems to have mostly subsided. Soy used to be pushed as one of the best alternatives to dairy, but some studies have now discovered too much soy might

have negative effects on female fertility
and reproductive development.

And despite all of this talk about food and
the conflicting arguments about what we
should eat and how we should eat it, more
of us are removed from the genesis of our
food than ever before. In my family, I'm
part of the first generation who did not
grow up on a farm. Think about that. But I
know where milk and eggs come from. I've
actually been to a farm. Spoken to farmers.

I also know what a chicken looks like before
it hits my plate—unlike a friend of mine in
high school. After I gave her a recipe that
called for cubed chicken, she phoned me
when she couldn't find it at the grocery
store. She actually thought chicken came
cubed. She didn't realize you had to cut it
into cubes. Some of you might be rolling
your eyes, but she was a smart girl. And I'll
bet she didn't know where beef tenderloin
came from either.

Why does it matter that we know? So we
can make sure we can bless the origins of
our food and understand how it connects
us to the people and land involved in it.

But it's also so we can keep an eye on how our food is being altered in the sometimes-crazy food industry.

Mother Nature isn't too fond of changes to the natural order. Like us, plants and animals were designed perfectly and uniquely. They have their own needs for nourishment to help them remain in their most natural state.

Think of all the over-bred turkeys for Thanksgiving. I remember my mom, who recalls going to a cousin's farm that raised turkeys back in the day, telling me many of them are now bred with such large breasts that they literally can't stand up without falling over. They can't even mate naturally anymore. Why is this happening? Because a bunch of "food experts" started telling us white meat was better for us than dark meat, when apparently the differences are minimal. Now we've created bigger-breasted turkeys because we want to eat more white meat than dark, and it's harming the natural order. That's not good.

What if someone or something decided to alter us that way? I don't think this is what the Universe had in mind for us.

Are you feeling a little depressed after reading all this? You're not alone. Folks, we have a lot of stories going on about food. And a lot of issues to work through because of them.

When in the hell did eating get so complicated?

Maybe it's always been this complicated.

Doesn't it strike you as ironic that in the Christian creation story Adam and Eve were kicked out of the Garden of Eden for *eating*?

But this isn't the only creation myth involving food. With the Yoruba, the story includes a five-toed chicken, some dirt, and a palm nut. Other stories involve the egg, while many indigenous myths feature corn. Most of these stories involve a life-altering conflict and some really interesting plot twists like the first people's bodies being cut up or torn apart and then buried in the ground or thrown into the sea to create all sorts of animal species and trees and plants for us to eat. *Yum.*

In those stories, the point is that if a god or goddess or God or deity (or whatever you want to call it) was going to create a planet and a bunch of humans, something had to be available for dinner, right? Even though many people now largely see these myths as symbolic in the face of evolution— something we don't need to debate for our purposes here—it doesn't change the fact that we've been selecting foods and eating meals since the dawn of time.

But food no longer seems to be viewed as the vital source of nourishment that gave rise to all these myths.

If you're reading this, you want to have a new relationship with food. Maybe it's something you've struggled with all of your life. Maybe it's something that's just popped up out of nowhere. Maybe you're feeling as conflicted and confused by the profusion of stories and unsure of where it leaves you.

Don't worry. Your goddess woman self has plans for you. She wants you to reclaim your birthright: a divine partnership with food, your own personal goddess menu.

Are you ready?

Let's dig in.

CHAPTER 2

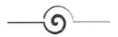

YOUR MAJOR BREAKDOWN(S) WITH FOOD

As we've discussed in the other *Goddess Guides*, we are all born fully wired to our goddess natures. No baby carries stories about food—they accept it, gladly, as a source of nourishment. They have no self-consciousness about their bodies, whether they have the adorable chubby thighs of infancy or the rail-thin bodies of some busy and growing toddlers.

And yet that innate wiring gets screwed up the longer we're in the world. People make hurtful comments. They start trying to rewire you to their stories (either because they think it's loving or because they don't believe you're good enough as you are). Maybe you allow it; maybe you don't see another choice. Maybe you even rewire yourself to their story to get love, approval, affection, etc. Things get a little messed up. You get separated from your goddess woman self. You stop seeing eating food as something simple and necessary and enjoyable.

The process really *is* simple. Food is *designed* (by the Universe or God or the Divine or whatever you consider the source of life) to nourish our goddess woman bodies while we're alive, and it's cultivated by humans to ensure we have enough of it (ideally).

But the stories we carry about food stand in the way of this divine partnership. And one of the major ones plaguing most of us women is body image. Now, *Goddesses Are Sexy* discusses reclaiming a loving self-image, and as such it's a wonderful sister guide to this one if this is something you're struggling with. In this guide, however, we're going to focus on what it means to eat as a goddess woman fully aligned with our divine formula:

Goddess+Food=Nourishment

And we need to start with the first major breakdown between our sense of self and food.

As we've discussed, girls are starting to diet at younger ages. They're being taught that anything more or less than the perfect weight is not okay, and that food is essentially the enemy.

We're going to start off by considering the girl who has been taught her body is too large, that she shouldn't eat so much. This is the so-called big-boned girl whose parents don't allow her to eat carbs as a strategy to make her look less large for her age, or less large period; the girl who isn't allowed to eat cheese or bread because her mom is worried she might get fat young because that's what happened to her at that age; the girl whose parents take her to a dietician and then serve her extra vegetables when her other siblings get to eat everything on the table; one who has her lunch consistently stolen at school by thin-girl bullies because they say she's too fat to need it.

My own first major breakdown with food fits into this category.

Dieting was considered normal in my own all-girls high school, and I remember being mocked for being a little larger than the so-called popular girls and for not eating rice cakes for lunch.

Their jabs at my then size-ten body made an impression, but the most painful jab came from my mother. My soul must have taken a snapshot that day because I remember it vividly: what room we were in, the fact that I was a junior in high school, and that she was wearing a white nightgown when it happened. She looked at me and said, "What's happened to my daughter? The one who used to be skinny?"

I was devastated. *Dev-a-stated.* If you've ever had anyone you love say something like that to you, you know what I mean.

It was all the more upsetting because my mom knew I couldn't exercise anymore. Long story short, I broke my hip as a freshman and was told I'd never walk again. The good news was that I did walk again, but one of the outcomes of the medical condition was that I couldn't (at the time) do any more of the sports I loved like running or basketball. I could only walk, and even then not much or my hip would start hurting. I hated not being able to do the things I used to. I hated the changes in my body.

Though I did give in to the pull to throw up on a few occasions, my goddess woman self was clearly working overtime because I knew doing it consistently would hurt my body. I'd read about the effects of anorexia and bulimia in biology class since eating disorders were a big problem in my high school and often discussed. As a student counselor, I even listened to other girls who were plagued by the issue. Honestly, I was also terrified my mom would find out and punish me. I can appreciate the mixed blessing in that parenting style now.

But maybe you had a different story going on. Maybe you were considered too thin and were made fun of because of it. One of my sisters was called "chicken legs," while another was called "Ethiopia" as a baby and toddler because she looked so underweight for her height. This is the girl whose parents worry endlessly about her because she can never put on any weight despite how much they encourage her to eat; the one whose teachers drop hints that she might have an eating disorder; the one who is bullied by other girls for being a "skinny bitch."

I'm also going to throw out the possibility that your major breakdown with food and your self-image didn't have anything to do with weight. Perhaps it had something to do with the people who raised you, be it parents or a caregiver. Maybe they didn't care whether you were fed. They didn't buy groceries, and you were always hungry. They didn't cook for you, so you had to forage for yourself. Your take-away was that you didn't matter, that you were nothing to the people who were supposed to love you and take care of you. And so food is another source of your lack of self-worth when it comes to love and relationships with those closest to you. This is the kid who is too hungry to focus in class and because of it doesn't get good grades; the one who doesn't go out for sports because it burns too many calories.

Or maybe your parents overfed you or were always forcing food on you as a way of making up for their perceived failings. Perhaps it was their way of trying to show their love for you because they didn't see you very much because they were working or traveling, or because they didn't have shared custody after the divorce. You were taught you had to prove your love to them by eating. You started to believe something was wrong with you; or that you were a bad girl when you protested eating was something they were trying to force on you. You might also have started believing you had no personal power of your own, something discussed at greater length in *Goddesses Decide*. This is the kid who walks around perpetually full or stuffed, especially after being with their parent, the kid who has trouble naturally moving through the day or doing anything physical because her body is always trying to digest what she has consumed.

How about we take a moment to think back on your life growing up so we can identify the first major breakdown(s) and tell it to take a hike?

Reclaiming Practice Intro

As goddess women, we're equipped with a tool I love to call "The Blaster." This baby is a set of phrases power-packed with energy to blast out the stories that have invaded your life and overtaken the natural divine formulas you were born with. If you're already familiar with this tool, go on and get going. First-timers, hang with me a bit as I explain a little more.

These reclaiming practices tackle your beliefs head on, which make up your story. Then bit by bit, we blast them out. We don't need or want this junk obscuring our goddess woman selves any more or being the place from which we make decisions. Think of it as computer code. We're rewiring our systems back to our goddess woman selves before all the stories overrode our perfect original programming.

And this even goes for the stories we perceive are positive. This might seem counterintuitive, but here's the thing: we may still be seeing them with our old glasses and not our stylish new goddess shades. I know this was true for me. What I thought was "good" or "fine" turned out not to be very goddess-like. But we also do this to wipe the slate completely clean so there isn't anything between you and your goddess nature. This ensures it's a complete reset. Make sense?

Personally, I like to say these phrases out loud because speaking them with one's voice amplifies our commitment to blasting them out, especially when we're starting out on our goddess journey.

If you find yourself coughing or "losing your voice," it's totally normal. Why? Because those stories have been clogging your pipes, so to speak. You'll know when you need to say something more than once. And once you know "The Blaster" by heart, your goddess self will show you what other stories you need to delete. The important thing is to feel empowered over the stories in your life and reclaim your full goddess nature.

Reclaiming Practice #1:

Blasting Out the Breakdowns

I'll bet your goddess self is helping you remember your first hurtful breakdown with food. Take a minute and let the images come to mind. Perhaps you're seeing no more than a flicker of a memory, or maybe it's an entire movie reel. Let that humdinger come to you, and if you find yourself getting emotional, don't worry. That's totally normal. This kind of crap hurts, even if it happened a while ago. Don't overthink it. Allow more details to surface so you can let them all go.

And if you're angry, that's okay. You have every right to be. The question is: do you want to keep being angry? Your goddess self is kindly suggesting there's a happier way for you, and she's ready to guide you.

If you have more than one story that you remember, I'd recommend taking them one at a time so you can be fully present to the story, the people involved, and all the feelings you have around it.

We're going to clear these stories by the categories my goddess self guided me to share here. Find the one(s) that you feel resonates the most with you and repeat after me:

If your story is about being fat...

All of the comments people have made about my

weight, I transmute, clear, and delete them.

Everywhere I started to believe I was fat (and ridiculed myself for it), I transmute, clear, and delete it.

All of the reasons I was told it was because of food, I transmute, clear, and delete them.

All of the punishments I was given for eating, I transmute, clear, and delete them.

All of the times I was made to eat different foods or diet because I was considered fat or an over-eater, I transmute, clear, and delete them.

All of the reasons I couldn't eat like a normal kid, I transmute, clear, and delete them.

All of the encouragement I was given (from myself or others) to watch what I ate and what I weighed, I transmute, clear, and delete it.

All of the times I was shamed, bullied, or mocked, I transmute, clear, and delete them.

All of the worries leveled at me (from myself or others) about my health, well-being, or lack of exercise, I transmute, clear, and delete them.

All of my beliefs that it's totally unfair, I transmute, clear, and delete them.

All of the ways it's affected my life, I transmute, clear, and delete them.

All of the shame, anger, and sadness it made me feel, I transmute, clear, and delete them.

Any remaining stories about me and food, I transmute, clear, and delete them.

If your story is about being too skinny...

All of the comments people have made about my weight, I transmute, clear, and delete them.

All of the times I was told something was wrong with me, I transmute, clear, and delete them.

All of the times I was told I didn't eat enough, I transmute, clear, and delete them.

All of the times I had to reassure myself (and others) that I ate plenty, but it just wouldn't stick to my bones, I transmute, clear, and delete them.

All of the reasons food was considered the problem for me, I transmute, clear, and delete them.

All of the worries people had about my health or well-being or over-stimulation, I transmute, clear, and delete them.

All of the ways it affected my life, I transmute, clear, and delete them.

All of the shame, anger, and sadness it made me feel, I transmute, clear, and delete them.

Any remaining stories about me and food, I transmute, clear, and delete them.

If your story is about not being fed...

All of the reasons no one cared about feeding me, I transmute, clear, and delete them.

All of the reasons no one cared about cooking for me, I transmute, clear, and delete them.

All of the reasons no one ever got groceries so I could eat, I transmute, clear, and delete them.

All of my guardians' excuses for why there wasn't food or money to buy food, I transmute, clear, and delete them.

All of the ways I had to fend for myself, I transmute, clear, and delete them.

All of the ways I couldn't fend for myself, I transmute, clear, and delete them.

All of the times I went hungry, I transmute, clear, and delete them.

All of the times I got light-headed or sick or couldn't focus, I transmute, clear, and delete them.

All of the ways it affected my life, I transmute, clear, and delete them.

All of the shame, anger, and sadness I have that this happened to me, I transmute, clear, and delete them.

Any remaining stories about me and food, I transmute, clear, and delete them.

If your story is about food being pushed on you...

All of the times I had food forced on me, I transmute, clear, and delete them.

All of the reasons it was forced on me, I transmute, clear, and delete them.

All of the times I didn't say no when I wanted to,

I transmute, clear, and delete them.

All of the reasons I didn't feel I could say no, I transmute, clear, and delete them.

All of the times I did say no and felt bad about it, I transmute, clear, and delete them.

All of the reasons I couldn't stop this cycle or end this story, I transmute, clear, and delete them.

All of the ways I felt sick or disgusted with myself, I transmute, clear, and delete them.

All of the ways it affected my life, I transmute, clear, and delete them.

All of the shame, anger, and sadness I have that this happened to me, I transmute, clear, and delete them.

Any remaining stories about me and food, I transmute, clear, and delete them.

Whew! Let's take a breath, shall we? There are a lot of feelings rising up, aren't there? If your throat or chest feels tight or your head is hurting, just keep breathing. Can you feel the first shaft of light from your goddess woman self?

Okay, let's put our hands on our hearts for a minute. Take another cleansing breath and just imagine all of that crap flying out of you like black smoke. It can't stay inside you anymore. It's time for it to go. Repeat after me when you're feeling a little calmer.

*I love and accept myself, exactly as
I was then and as I am now.*

Can you hear your heartbeat? You can listen for it. That's your beautiful heart, the one that's been holding all this hurt and anger. Your heart is transforming too.

How about we let go of the people involved in this story? Here's a little thing about forgiveness. It's really liberating, but when it comes to the people who have hurt us the most, it can be hard as hell to forgive them. It's taken me years to forgive someone who's starred in my major breakdowns. You know, the ones that feel like they'll stick in your mind *forever*.

But if you want to start today, let's give it a shot. Your goddess self is pushing up her sleeves, ready to dive in with you. If you're not ready yet, don't worry about it. Just skip on ahead. No one is forcing forgiveness or pushing forgiveness on you. It's always your choice.

If you'd like to continue, take a moment to bring to mind the main character(s) in your story. Maybe this person(s) is still in your life. Maybe he or she isn't. Maybe you got tag-teamed. Just take the characters in your story one at a time. Repeat after me:

X (Name), I don't know why you said what you did or why you treated me like that. It wasn't right. It was mean and hurtful, and I deserved better. I don't want to feel like this anymore, either about you or myself. I forgive you and my part in this story. I am willing to let it go. Mostly. Okay, all the way. Right now. I'm a goddess and this is how I roll.

Congratulations, goddess woman! You just got your first taste of epic freedom.

And we're just getting started.

CHAPTER 3

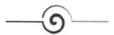

SAYING GOODBYE TO YOUR CURRENT RELATIONSHIP WITH FOOD

The way you treat yourself with food is an expression of your relationship with yourself and your life.

Read that again. It bears repetition.

So, what does this mean in practice?

When you are starving yourself, you are feeling starved in life. Or you feel like you *should* be starving. You are denying yourself the very nourishment inherent in our divine formula because of all the stories you're carrying about yourself and how things are going for you; maybe it's your way of seeking control in a life that feels very out of balance.

When you are overeating or bingeing, you are seeking something *more* because you're being denied somewhere or by someone, maybe even yourself. You are gorging yourself because you're so empty of what you truly need. Again, because of the stories you have going on.

What's the need in both cases?

Love. Pure and simple. The expression of that love in this case is nourishment. The kind that comes from giving ourselves what we need.

Oh, shit, I can hear some of you saying. *It is.*

Those of you who have been keeping food journals or working on this issue personally have likely been facing this bugaboo down for a while now. Perhaps you've already identified the sources for your particular struggle, whether it's the shame you feel about your body; and/or a lack of love, acceptance, and appreciation for your goddess woman self; and/or that starving yourself or overeating is the way you handle uncomfortable emotions and stress. It likely dates back to those major breakdowns we just discussed.

Maybe your current relationship is so troubling for you, it's the Goliath in your life—a giant you feel you can't possibly defeat.

The thing is, this is not about winning—you need food and always will. Rather, it's about aligning your needs with your goddess nature and allowing her to guide you in filling them. Once you've reconnected with the divine formula, the rest will fall into place. You'll be back to seeing food as nourishment for your body instead of the source of *your* personal nourishment.

You're likely reading this because you're not happy with your current food relationship, but in order to change that relationship, we must first understand it. So it's time to put on some big goddess shoes (pick a pair in your mind; mine are orange heels with a black stripe up the back) and face down your current relationship with food. We all have one; how we interact with food is how we interact with ourselves and life. Are you ready to be balls-out honest with yourself? Because honesty is the only way we can take responsibility for the current decisions we're making so we can make changes.

This is vulnerable stuff, right? How about I go first? Sometimes it's hard to get started on our own or take that first step, so seeing someone else do it can be helpful and empowering. By going first, I'm trying to give you an example of how you might go about it. Of course, if your goddess self wants you to do the exercise somewhat differently, listen to her. She's always the one who knows best.

Okay, here goes...

I sometimes overeat.

My mom used to say I was like my dad. He overeats too. And when she said it, there was a little shame thrown in. Okay, you've got the setup now. Mom says I'm like Dad, not her. (Her story was she often didn't eat because she forgot while running errands and taking care of kids.) Blah blah. We're all playing a part in a sucky story. But I'm not a kid anymore, and my story continues; I take responsibility for it now.

The thing is I love food, and sometimes I

just don't want to stop. Sure, I occasionally feel twinges from old stories—things about cleaning my plate (or others') and not wasting food. But there is also this other story about the food being so good in the moment that it will never be as good again. Are you laughing a little?

Cue the problem of being a foodie *for me*. I love to cook and had a brief stint working in an award-winning restaurant, followed by a year-long position as a private chef, while I was going to graduate school. I see cooking as an act of creation, and it's as powerful and exciting as writing a book or planting in my garden. There's a beauty to it, an art even. Because I love to be all food-alchemist-like, I rarely use a recipe. I like to say I got the gift from my grandmother, but I can sense when certain foods are going to work together. I like to think it's because there's always been a part of me connected to my intuitive goddess nature through food.

It's not just my own cooking I savor. If I end up being served something absolutely scrumptious when I go out to a restaurant, I want to eat it all.

Then there's the whole stress eating. Yep. I do it. I used to do it a lot more than I do now because I've been clearing my stories for a while. I remember joking with colleagues when I used to work corporate that our three main food groups for when we were crashing on a major deadline were wine, chocolate, and cookies. And I used to bring in enough cookies to feed everyone on the team. I fed people constantly during the process to help them feel like I cared about them and appreciated everything they were doing.

Are you wondering if I still have moments when I want to reward myself with food? Yep! Like if I finish writing this chapter, I can have something special. But I'm on to that story too, and I can clear it when it comes. Of course, if I'm really hungry, that's a different story. I eat.

I still find myself eating potato chips in bulk—sometimes even after I've had dinner. It's like I crave the taste of them, and they never disappoint.

Wondering if I do comfort food? Yep. I find myself gravitating toward cooking or eating foods my grandmother would make when I was a kid, things like fried chicken and mashed potatoes. The other day I even caught myself wanting to ask my BFF what her favorite meal was as a way of trying to make her feel better after an emotionally challenging day. Luckily, she gets the whole "story" thing, so when I told her, she said, "You don't have to do that. Your presence is enough." That's the power of connection, something we'll talk about later.

I sometimes forget to eat when I'm really into my writing, and then it's like I could eat my arm, I am so hungry. I totally overeat in those moments because it's like I need to fill up the hole in there.

One thing I don't do is starve myself... And here's why. When I was working in Latin America in my mid-twenties, I developed a tropical illness and contracted parasites (ones that were drug-resistant). Everything I ate made me violently sick, and suddenly food was poison to my body. I lost twenty pounds in ten days. The weight loss was so pronounced that infectious disease doctors thought I had cancer on two occasions (I didn't, thankfully).

However, my body was ravaged by the illness and the parasites for the course of nine months. I couldn't work and went on workman's comp. It was terrifying and life-altering. I became so thin that I was downright fragile. I had trouble walking around the block, something I tried to do to keep the blood circulating, especially given the kind of medicine I was taking to fight the parasites. My food choices narrowed to small, easily digestible portions of lamb, chicken, and beef, and vegetables.

Even then, my belly would bloat after eating; sometimes I looked like I was five months pregnant. My enlarged abdomen would press into my lungs and cut off my airflow. I'd have trouble breathing and had to fight the panic simmering underneath the surface.

But one thing I clearly remember is feeling starved. *Constantly.*

I would look at food and want to eat it, but I couldn't. And that aching feeling, that hunger was a constant companion for me.

I still dance with wanting to make sure I have enough food around. Sure, some of that comes from traveling to war-torn countries that didn't always have a lot of food. I remember taking three weeks of health food bars, beef jerky, nuts, and dried fruit with me on a trip to Eastern Congo. And I went through all of it because there either wasn't enough food available or it wasn't safe to seek it out.

But deep down, I know there's still a little unhealed part of me that is worried about starving again. Even though I know there is no way that's ever going to happen. I'm going to clear that story the whole way and be free of its dark whispers. I've come so far from the trauma that a long-term illness can leave in its wake.

All of this is to say, I have things I'm still working on, stories I'm still clearing *all the way*. I'm not perfect, but I love myself however I am. I'm a goddess woman in progress.

You are too.

RECLAIMING PRACTICE #2:
Cleaning Out the Cupboard

I want to encourage those of you who journal

to write your own story, much like I just did with mine. If you're not someone who likes to write, no worries. Just sit back a bit and let the images come up. Or if you've written this story a million times and are sick of it, don't worry. Our Goddess Blaster is super-charged to help free you of these old patterns.

Let's start off by considering some questions:

What is your current relationship with food?

Is it the enemy? Is it your friend? Are you neutral about it?

Do you find yourself wishing you didn't have to eat or that you could eat all the time and not get fat? Do you wish you could afford to eat healthier? Organic fruits and vegetables are so expensive, right? Or do you find yourself wishing you didn't eat out all the time? Maybe you eat fast food more often than you would like because you're too busy to cook at home?

Once you've written about (or brought to mind) your current story about food, we're going to do a clearing exercise focused on the most common behaviors associated with straying from the divine formula (*Goddess+Food=Nourishment*): starving, dieting, and overeating and bingeing. Choose whichever behaviors you relate to most. Or focus on something else, from your own personal experience. (I don't mean for these categories to be taken as the sum total of all possible food-related behaviors.)

If you've experienced (or are experiencing) more than just one story, go ahead and clear the others too. This way you'll make sure there are no latent or hidden stories inside you. If they surface later, you know how to clear them then. It's easy.

Will there be emotion with this reclaiming practice? Of course! We're talking about feeling deep levels of personal denial and emptiness here. But this is another step toward feeling free—and nourished.

Let's go general first. Repeat after me:

All of the stories I have about food, I transmute, delete, and clear them.

All of the sources I learned them from, I trans-mute, delete, and clear them.

All of the patterns I have about food, I trans-mute, delete, and clear them.

Everything I think and feel when I see food, I transmute, delete, and clear it.

Whatever my relationship with food is right now, I transmute, delete, and clear it.

Whatever my relationship with food was, I transmute, delete, and clear it.

All of the reasons I'm not connected to the divine formula about food anymore, I transmute, delete, and clear them.

If you've starved yourself or consistently deny yourself food, repeat after me:

Everything driving me to starve myself or not eat, I transmute, delete, and clear it.

All of the reasons I don't eat or want to eat, I transmute, delete, and clear them.

All of the reasons I want to eat but won't let myself, I transmute, delete, and clear them.

All of the reasons I've accepted going hungry or feeling hungry, I transmute, delete, and clear them.

All of the times I wanted something other than food and wouldn't give it to myself, I transmute, delete, and clear them.

All of the ways I'm punishing myself, I transmute, delete, and clear them.

All of the energy I've poured into chasing a certain weight, I transmute, delete, and clear it.

Everywhere I believe this behavior is serving me or working for me, I transmute, delete, and clear it.

Everywhere I know it's wrong or I'm hurting myself, I transmute, delete, and clear it.

All of the people I'm listening to who validate this story, I transmute, delete, and clear them (not them physically, only their role).

All of the shame and hurt keeping me locked into this pattern, I transmute, delete, and clear it.

If you diet consistently, repeat after me:

All of the reasons I diet, I transmute, delete, and clear them.

All of the diet crazes I follow or have followed, and my reasons for doing so, I transmute, delete, and clear them.

All of the energy I've poured into chasing a certain weight, I transmute, delete, and clear it.

All of the fear and shame I feel because it never seems to work or produce lasting effects, I transmute, delete, and clear it.

All of the reasons I can't stop, I transmute, delete, and clear them.

All of the people I'm listening to who validate this story, I transmute, delete, and clear them (not them physically, only their role).

If you binge or consistently find yourself overeating, repeat after me:

All of the reasons I overeat or binge, I transmute, delete, and clear them.

All of the reasons I can't stop myself from eating, I transmute, delete, and clear them.

All of the reasons I don't want to stop, I transmute, delete, and clear them.

All of the reasons I want to stop but can't, I transmute, delete, and clear them.

The shame I feel because I know better and I do it anyway, I transmute, delete, and clear it.

The way I feel bloated or sick or horrible afterward, I transmute, delete, and clear it.

Everything I'm trying to fill, I transmute, delete, and clear it.

All of the reasons it's never enough, I transmute, delete, and clear them.

All of the people I'm listening to who validate this story, I transmute, delete, and clear them (not them physically, only their role).

Okay, let's all take some deep breaths. Memories of your relationship with food (like our breakdown moments) might be flashing into your mind as well as all the feelings associated with them. Maybe the shame is coming up too, making you want to hide or flee. Take a minute and let whatever wants to come on up do so. It's ready to fly out of you because you're ready to fly, goddess woman. Put your hand on your heart and take another deep breath. You're doing great! Stay with me.

RECLAIMING PRACTICE #3:
General Clearing

Is there anything that seems to be linger-ing, like it's attached to the bumper of your car and just won't let go? Let your goddess nature guide you through whatever wants to come up.

Repeat after me:

Everywhere I X (Name that behavior!), I trans-mute and clear it.

All of the reasons I X, I transmute and clear them.

All of the places I learned this behavior, I trans-mute and clear them.

All of the people involved, I transmute and clear them (not them physically, only their role).

All of the reasons X seems to plague me, I trans-mute and clear them.

All of the reasons I can't love myself in the moment or at all, I transmute and clear them.

Everywhere I feel all this pressure, I transmute and clear it.

All of the ways I feel like I don't measure up, I transmute and clear them.

All of the reasons I can't stop doing X, I transmute and clear them.

Everything I'm holding onto right now about X, I transmute and clear them.

Now I invite all of you to join me to clear stories we have in common because of these patterns about food.

Everywhere I'm carrying shame and hurt and negative thoughts and feelings about myself, I transmute, delete, and clear it.

Everywhere I might hate myself and all the reasons, I transmute, delete, and clear it.

Everywhere I wish I were different, looked different, walked different, acted different, was different, I transmute, delete, and clear it.

Everywhere I wish other people would help me, I transmute, delete, and clear it.

Everywhere this is a call for love, attention, or comfort, I transmute, delete, and clear it.

Everywhere I wish this would all be done and I could just be happy and eat like a "normal" person, I transmute, delete, and clear it.

Take a breath, goddess woman. You're doing great. Do you still have your hand on your heart? Listen for your heartbeat and take another deep breath. Repeat after me:

I love and accept myself.

Just as I am right now.

Regardless of all of my perceived faults (by myself and others), which I hereby delete and transmute.

I am a goddess woman, and I can create a new relationship with food, one that nourishes my goddess woman self.

You bet you can! Ready for one of our Goddess Declarations?

GODDESS DECLARATION
Creating YOUR Goddess Relationship with Food

That's right. Your new relationship with food is *yours* to choose and create as you desire. The old one is on its way out. Sure, you might still feel tugs in the old direction, mostly in the beginning as you're anchoring in this new goddess woman relationship. When that happens, get your Goddess Blaster out and go to town. If you end up going back to that old relationship for a moment or a day or a week or a month, you can use this same tool to free yourself of any anger or frustration you feel, reaffirming the love you feel for yourself and for this declaration. The point is to not be hard on yourself because that's just feeding the old relationship, right? When you can see your actions with compassionate and loving eyes, you leap back to your true goddess woman nature.

Repeat after me:

I hereby declare that I want a new relationship with food, one that serves my goddess woman self and body. I won't let anything get in the way—not even me.

I am willing to see food in a new light and interact with it in a new light. I am willing to see it as nourishment for this beautiful and sexy body I have. I am willing to enjoy my personal goddess menu every day, the one my goddess self guides me toward. She's my best friend when it comes to helping me choose the best menu for me—not anyone else.

I am willing to listen to my goddess self until this new relationship is so much a part of me, I don't even think about it anymore. It just is. It's how I roll.

I am willing to change any beliefs or behaviors I have around food and remove all toxic influences, even ones coming from people I love and care about.

I am willing to love food again in its purest form and let it nourish me like it was designed to.

And I do all of this because I love myself. Most of all.

Yay! You did it. Take a deep breath and give yourself a high five or pat on the back. That pledge just changed your whole relationship with food.

Now that you've decided to leave your old relationship with food in the past, let's take steps to ensure it stays there.

CHAPTER 4

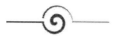

THE ROOTS AND THE RECLAIMING: FLASH ROUND

Let's keep turning the pages of your storybook, goddess woman.

You've been eating for a long while now, so there are lots of memories and experiences filling up that storybook. Somewhere along the way, your old relationship with food took root. Note the use of the world "old." That's done, it ended when you made a commitment to a new relationship with food.

But here's the thing about roots—if you don't pull all of them up, another weed might spring to life. We're going to dig way down to the sources of those old stories to make sure we get *all* the roots. Put on your goddess shoes (mine today are two-inch turquoise heels with diamonds on the tips). This is probably going to require major goddess woman honesty and heart. If you have a journal, you might want to jot some ideas down as they come to you or write your own story when you finish reading here.

We're going to do what I'll call a Flash Round. I'm going to throw out a whole bunch of possible story nudges to help those old memories surface, and then I'm going to share my story as a sort of template before you either write or contemplate your own story. (If your parents didn't raise you, please change the questions to best fit your life experience.) The next step is to use our Goddess Blaster to help us further reset our goddess woman selves back to our divine formula. Prepare to say *sayonara* to a whole bunch of stories in rapid, goddess-like fashion.

Story Nudges: Let's start with when you were young. What was eating like for you then? Were you a happy kid who couldn't wait to eat? One who loved to eat watermelon and spit the seeds out, giggling all the while? Or were you a picky eater? One who never liked anything your parent(s) served you? What was the nature of your food? Was it home-cooked, takeout, fast food, or restaurant style?

My Answer: I loved to eat and am grateful to both my mom and my maternal grandma for making food mostly a happy place. They were both great cooks. Being from the Midwest and originally from the farm, our family ate a good breakfast in the morning, usually eggs, French toast, or pancakes with bacon, sausage, and the occasional fruit. Lunch was a simple sandwich, chips, and maybe an apple. After homework we could have a cookie from the cookie jar. For dinner, we had a meat, a starch (usually potatoes), and a vegetable for dinner. We usually had a dessert in the form of a cake or a pie. Our food was simple without a lot of spices, and we didn't have much fresh vegetables except in the summertime.

Ironically, it was because we didn't have a lot of money that we ate almost exclusively home-cooked meals. Fast food was a rare treat—and one we begged for since "all the other kids" got to eat it. Happy Meals at McDonald's were new at the time and a huge deal back then (and let's take a minute to appreciate that phrase, Happy Meal—talk about positive association). Our family only went to a restaurant for things like the baptism of a new baby in our family or First Communion, and these occasions were always tinged with stress about money: we could only order water; we couldn't order anything expensive; and in some cases we even shared a plate.

Your Answer: Fill it in mentally or physically by writing it down.

Goddess Blaster:

All of my stories around food when I was a kid, I transmute, clear, and delete them.

All of the reasons I didn't like eating, I transmute, clear, and delete them.

Anywhere food wasn't happy, I transmute, clear, and delete them.

All of the kinds of food or places to eat that didn't work for me, I transmute, clear, and delete them.

All of the negative associations here, I transmute,

clear, and delete them.

Story Nudges: Who cooked for you? Was one or more of the people who raised you a good cook? Were the women in your family the only ones who cooked or did some of the men too, including your dad if he was around? Were you included in the cooking and was this a happy place for you or a chore?

My Answer: As I said above, my mom was a great cook and did so exclusively in our household. I loved to cook, and I was often included as a helper in making meals, beginning when I was very young. I have happy memories of being offered a batter-coated beater and licking it with delight. Over time, I ended up taking on a large part of the cooking, especially when my mom had to pick up siblings at after-school events like soccer or gymnastics. I was able to explore new recipes, which gave me a new sense of accomplishment and freedom. But my most precious memories of cooking as a child and young adult were from the summers I spent alone with my grandmother. I had her all to myself, and for a kid who was one of six children, it was a rare and magical time to be the center of one person's attention and love.

But there was always a clear gender divide in the kitchen. Only women cooked, and I remember being angry that all of the men got to sit in front of the TV watching football (something I love too) while I had to cook *for them* in the kitchen. Why did they get to sit around while I was working? It didn't seem fair that it was only because they were men. My brothers broke this gender mold by helping in the kitchen, but this experience in my childhood had a profound effect on me.

Your Answer: Take a moment to think about your story here. There's no rush. Let it surface in your mind or write it down.

Goddess Blaster:

All of the stories I have around who cooked when I was growing up, I transmute, clear, and delete them.

All of the reasons these aren't happy memories, I transmute, clear, and delete them.

All of the resentment I felt when X (Name) fed

me or tried to feed me, I transmute, clear, and delete it.

Everything I took away from these experiences about food, cooking, and my very self, I transmute, clear, and delete it.

All of the times I wanted something different or someone who could cook better, I transmute, clear, and delete them.

Everything else that wants to be released, I transmute, clear, and delete it.

Story Nudges: Was there enough (or more than enough) food to go around? Who did the shopping? Did someone clip coupons and read the grocery store sale ads? Was your pantry well-stocked or did your parent(s) live paycheck to paycheck? Did you consume generic food products or the best-of-the-best?

My Answer: Since I'm from a big family that didn't have much money, like I've mentioned before, food was sometimes stretched. Sauces were thinned down, and meat was sometimes sparse in soups or stews. If I wanted a second helping, I learned to eat fast so I could pile on more mashed potatoes before my younger brother, for example. And my mom often ate less so we could have more.

She was also a master at using coupons and shopping the sales. We often used generic or "club" products, not name brands. We had a big freezer in the garage, so she would buy meat when it was on sale and stock it away until we needed it.

I remember her telling this story about being on the church council when another member wanted to increase the priest's monthly food allowance to something she considered very high. She shocked them by saying she fed our family of eight people on five hundred dollars a month. I also remember her saying she wished she could walk into the grocery store and buy whatever she wanted. I felt the same way and would look longingly at certain foods that struck my fancy that we couldn't afford.

Your Answer: What are you remembering? Let your goddess self show you, and if you're journaling, fill out the story there. And take a deep breath while you're at it.

Goddess Blaster:

All of my links between food and money, I transmute, clear, and delete them.

My beliefs that some brands or products are inferior to others, I transmute, clear, and delete them.

My beliefs that a stocked cupboard or pantry meant you were rich, I transmute, clear, and delete them.

All of the stories other people had around groceries that I took on—consciously or unconsciously—I transmute, clear, and delete them.

All of the reasons I didn't have enough food or what I wanted to eat, I transmute, clear, and delete them.

All of the times I still hold back on buying what I want or need at the grocery store, I transmute, clear, and delete them.

Everything else that needs to clear here, I transmute, clear, and delete it.

Story Nudges: What were you taught about food? Did your parent(s) or relatives teach you certain phrases about it? Were they pearls of wisdom or sayings laced with shame, like gluttony being a sin?

My Answer: Growing up, we often were told never to waste food, that whole "waste not, want not" saying. Starving children in Africa were mentioned—Ethiopia, specifically—as a way to encourage us to be grateful for the food we had. We ate everything on our plate, even if we were full. If we had leftovers, we ate them as well.

We were taught food was a precious gift. This stemmed from the desire not to waste money, sure, but it was more than that. Food was a celebration, and family reunions certainly showed that. The tables were always loaded with home-cooked, simple food.

While my grandma was teaching me how to cook, she was also teaching me to show love for my family by doing so. You made something special for someone if they were coming to visit or if it was their birthday. You got to pick your meal on that day, even steak, a treat.

I also remember hearing "a way to a man's

heart is through his stomach." I figured way back when that I had this covered. I was a great cook. I was frequently told I'd make a great wife.

People also used the phrase "champagne tastes on a beer budget" in my family a lot, especially when it came to food.

Another interesting story was about the supposed correlation between women not eating breakfast, especially when they were growing up, and later having miscarriages. I can't tell you the number of times I heard this story, mostly because one of my sisters didn't like to eat breakfast. All of the female members of my family can probably still cite X family member and her number of miscarriages off the tops of their heads.

Your Answer: Take a moment to let it come to you. Maybe close your eyes a minute and see what you remember. If you're writing, your journal is probably on fire by now, and that's a good thing.

Goddess Blaster:

All of the phrases about food I heard growing up,

I transmute, clear, and delete them.

All of the stories I was told about eating and food, I transmute, clear, and delete them.

Everywhere I took on these stories and made them my own, I transmute, clear, and delete it.

All of the so-called wisdom imparted to me, I transmute, clear, and delete it.

All of the ways it limited my actions or shamed me, I transmute, clear, and delete them.

All of the people attached to these stories, I transmute, clear, and delete them (don't worry, you aren't deleting them; you're only removing the power you gave them in your story).

Story Nudges: Was food used as a tool to reward, control, or punish you? Were you ever sent to bed without supper if you did something "bad" like talk back? Or spanked for not eating? Did anyone make you stay at the table until you finished your plate? Were you told you could have a treat or a snack if you were a "good" girl and did X thing? Did you observe the people who raised you giving themselves a treat after a long day or punishing themselves over food, like not eating when they were hungry?

My Answer: We often had a treat after we did our homework, something that continued as I got older. At any given meal, one or two siblings would usually get into trouble for not eating something on their plate or not finishing it, so there was some drama at the table, something I remember not enjoying.

As you may have read in *Goddesses Don't Do Drama*, my dad is an alcoholic. When he came home, he'd immediately start drinking. For a long time, I attributed this to how people rewarded themselves after enduring a long, hard day.

Your Answer: You know what to do here.

Goddess Blaster:

All of my memories of being punished with food, I transmute, clear, and delete them.

All of my memories of being rewarded with food, I transmute, clear, and delete them.

All of the reasons X (Name whoever comes to

mind) did this, I transmute, clear, and delete them.

All of the ways I started to link food and reward, control, or punishment, I transmute, clear, and delete them.

All of the times I've done the same to myself or someone else, I transmute, clear, and delete them.

All of the ways I'm playing out these patterns as an adult, I transmute, clear, and delete them.

Story Nudges: Were you one of the girls who were encouraged to start watching what you ate, e.g. dieting young? Did one of your parents or both diet so you had to follow suit and eat like they did? Did everyone eat something different? Or did you have someone constantly push food at you as a way of showing their love or dominance? Were you forced to eat when you didn't want to?

My Answer: I don't have any deep-seated stories here, but I remember having to eat a second holiday meal at my paternal grandparents' house. This grandmother wasn't a great cook, and their story with food was completely different than mine. It wasn't happy. I remember not wanting to go over there to eat; in fact, I didn't want to go period. My parents insisted I had to eat so I wouldn't hurt her feelings.

Your Answer: Your goddess self and you are on fire. Keep letting her show you what you need to remember.

Goddess Blaster:

All of the reasons X (Name whoever comes to mind) told me I had to watch what I ate, I transmute, clear, and delete them.

Everywhere my food intake was restricted, I transmute, clear, and delete it.

Everywhere my choices of what to eat were limited or controlled, I transmute, clear, and delete it.

Everywhere I had to eat what I was told to eat— even if I was full or not hungry—I transmute, clear, and delete it.

Story Nudges: What kinds of religious or spiritual stories were you told about food? Were any foods taboo or sacred, either for religious or cultural reasons? Were there any foods you didn't eat during certain times of the year? Was fasting part of your religious or spiritual experience? (Please note, I'm not making any suggestions, comments, or judgments about these traditions in and of themselves. This is about how *you* feel, and that's for you and your goddess self to decide. Trust me, if there's something that doesn't make you feel loved or peaceful, it's ready to go.)

My Answer: Since I grew up Catholic, we didn't eat meat on Fridays during Lent (and Ash Wednesday). We could only eat fish. We also weren't supposed to snack between main meals. I hated these days because we ended up eating things like fish sticks, which tasted gross to me at the time. I also didn't understand why meat wasn't okay on that one day of the week and fish was; the rule wasn't consistent and had no translation in my mind to being a good person.

When I learned in my Catholic school religion class that the whole fish thing came about because of a pope who was trying to support fishermen (something some people now claim isn't a true story), I was outraged. I didn't like that someone had used his power as a religious official to subvert my free will as a spiritual individual for no moral reason, especially since he was essentially proclaiming those who didn't follow the rule weren't good people. Thankfully, I grew up in a pretty open-minded family when it came to these kinds of religious dictates, so I wasn't forced to fall in line once I was old enough to make my own decision about it.

But that didn't put an end to all the talk about sin around food. Teachers and priests told me that I had to confess to a priest if I broke one of those rules during Lent. We were also encouraged to give up foods we especially loved during Lent, which I sometimes did—usually with a better attitude because it was my choice and not mandatory.

Your Answer: Take a moment and breathe. I have a feeling there are lots of you with stories that run deep here.

Goddess Blaster:

Everywhere food and religion are tied into my

story, I transmute, clear, and delete them.

Everywhere I still have spiritual or religious stories going on about food, I transmute, delete, and clear them.

All of the stories I was told about how following these rules made me a good person or more spiritual or religious or holy, I transmute, clear, and delete it.

All of the stories I was told about how eating something or eating it at a certain time was a sin or immoral, I transmute, clear, and delete them.

All of the people involved in these stories, I transmute, clear, and delete them (again, we're only deleting their role, not them).

All of the times I've passed these beliefs on to other people, I transmute, clear, and delete them.

All of these stories that don't serve me and my goddess woman self, I transmute, clear, and delete them.

Story Nudges: Do you recall any racial, cultural, or social comments being made about certain foods? Were there any restaurants you didn't patronize or foods you didn't eat due to racial, cultural, or social bias? Were you called any nasty names because of the foods you ate? Did people use offensive phrases about the food that was part of your heritage?

My Answer: Yep, and I was ashamed of that for a long time. Most of those comments came from my maternal grandpa, whom I dearly loved, who had a lot of racial prejudice. He was a really funny guy, so much of what he said in these terms was delivered as a joke or in a humorous tone. He said eating too much rice would make our eyes slant. He made negative comments about Polish food, something I remember from a cultural festival, and also about the Hispanics who ran the Mexican restaurant in my grandparents' small town in the Midwest— which he ate at and would take us to, by the way. He also referred to a type of nuts with a vile racial phrase (one I won't mention here), but one people still joke about in the family.

His comments always infuriated me, and I would often challenge him, especially as I grew older. Sometimes he'd laugh at me,

but other times I got reprimanded for talking back. Fighting with him about his views
about other people didn't change anything.
I was also told to respect him even if I didn't
like his views.

The only other thing this prompt brings
up for me is that I can remember discuss-
ing what rich people ate—crazy things like
caviar, for example, and paying a mint for
it—or talking about people who "ate at the
country club," ones who weren't considered
nice.

Your Answer: Keep going. You're doing
awesome. Do you have a story here? One
you need to clear? Take a breath with me.
Whew! Let's blast this crap out.

Goddess Blaster:

*All of the racial, cultural, or social phrases or
stories I have heard about people and food, I
transmute, clear, and delete them.*

*All of the stories I was told about how some peo-
ple's food was dirty or their restaurants weren't
clean, I transmute, clear, and delete them.*

All of the racial or cultural prejudices about

food or around food I've heard or picked up on, I transmute, clear, and delete them.

All of the times I participated in this talk or fought against it, I transmute, clear, and delete them.

All of the times X (Name whoever comes to mind) said X phrase or used X word, I transmute, clear, and delete them.

All of the horrible and offensive things people said about me and the food I ate, I transmute, clear, and delete them.

All of the shame and anger I felt at others because of what they said about the food I ate, I transmute, clear, and delete it.

Everyone I need to release, I transmute, clear, and delete them (again not them, but the power they have in your story).

All of the ways I started seeing myself differently and the food I ate because of their comments, I transmute, clear, and delete them.

All of the stories that are keeping me from being my full goddess woman self right now, I transmute, clear, and delete them.

Story Nudges: What were mealtimes like for you? Did you always eat at a set time when you were home, or was it free-form? Was the weekend schedule different? Did you eat as a family or do your own thing? Do you remember anyone stealing food off your plate, or did you steal it? Did you have to clean up or wipe down the table?

My Answer: We always ate dinner as a family at the table; we were never allowed to eat in front of the TV. Meals were considered family time, and we pretty much adhered to this even as we got older. My dad and mom sat at the heads of the table. I had my own chair, usually closest to the kitchen in case I needed to get up and grab something (which I just realized I still do and need to clear with the Goddess Blaster). We weren't allowed to leave the table until we were all finished eating; okay, sometimes there was one sibling who stayed at the table longer than the rest of us because she wouldn't eat her dinner.

If anyone tried to take food off my plate, I would take action, though usually in a way that wouldn't get me into trouble. Sometimes I would hunker down around my plate like I was guarding it, especially if we were eating something really good or special.

There were some routines that happened every dinner time. Usually my dad would ask us about our day because my mom already knew the details. I hated having to repeat my stories. We all took our plates and put them in the dishwasher. I remember lots of laughing and fighting. Sometimes siblings would be separated if they kept fighting.

Breakfast was usually consumed when it was ready, and we ate quickly during the week since we had school.

On the weekends, we usually ate right after 5 p.m. church. We made meals that accommodated that timeframe. If we went to mass Saturday night, we would make a feast on Sundays. It was a big spread, and we all sat down and enjoyed it. Again, we put our dishes in the dishwasher. I would usually help washing up pans, and for a long time, I did more cleaning as the oldest.

Your Answer: What about you? Take a

minute to remember. You're rocking this.

Goddess Blaster:

All of my associations between eating and family, I transmute, clear, and delete them.

All of the reasons I hated to eat as a family, I transmute, clear, and delete them.

All of my feelings about how we never ate together, I transmute, clear, and delete them.

All of my emotions about not having a family to sit down with, I transmute, clear, and delete them.

All of the links between eating at a set time or place, I transmute, clear, and delete them.

All of the links between eating and cleaning up, I transmute, clear, and delete them.

Everyone who is coming to mind in this story, I transmute, clear, and delete them.

Everything I took away about love, togetherness, and community, I transmute, clear, and delete them.

Everything I took away about what family meant or didn't mean, I transmute, clear, and delete them.

All of the other associations that want to go, I transmute, clear, and delete them.

Whoa! Do you feel like we've covered a lot of stories? You bet your ass we did. I told you the storybook you had about eating was sizeable! But it's not now because we just uprooted those old stories.

And this is just the start of uncovering all of the junk in the way of reconnecting you fully to our divine formula:

Goddess+Food=Nourishment

You might not feel like you're completely there yet, but we're well on our way.

CHAPTER 5

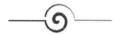

BLASTING CENTRAL

You've just made a huge dent in your old relationship with food. Take a breath. Give yourself a high five.

As I was writing this guide, one thing stood out, and that was how deep, complex, and layered our stories are about both our relationship with food and food itself. It was like a ball of cellophane wrap had gotten all tangled up.

Think of the divine formula as a perfect sheet of wrapping. But each of our personal stories adds an unnecessary sheet on top of the original. You'd think that would be enough, but no. We also have what I'll call a media blitz about food. According to one study I found through the U.S. National Institutes of Health, eleven out of nineteen commercials per hour are about food. And that's not even counting all of the billboards or online ads you get exposed to about this restaurant or this food. Let's throw these in as well; each one is another sheet. Then we have cooking shows and reality cooking shows. We're gorging on stories about food. Do you see where I'm going here? It's a big freaking ball of stories, and many of them are stuck to and tangled up with one another.

So, we're going to circle back to do a few more rounds of blasting, this time going even deeper and taking a more targeted approach. I want to take a final pass at blasting our current reasons for eating or not eating, because let's face it, your patterns here get activated every day—since your body needs sustenance every day. Talk about ingrained.

But we're also going to look at how all of our stories have affected what we currently eat. Again, this is intended to wipe the slate clean.

Then we're going to take a pass at all of the numbers we associate with food and eating.

They're everywhere, aren't they? On our food packaging, at the center of this and that diet, and the subject of a slew of promises about how much weight you might lose if you do x, y, and z. Many of us are playing a numbers game with food, and we need to clear that in order to reconnect to our divine formula.

I know it feels like we've been goddess blasting stories for a while now, but we need to address those before we can start eating like a goddess woman.

Reclaiming Practice #4:

Root Cause Blasting

How about we start by turning to some of the reasons we do what we do with food to make sure we've covered everything? Let's see if this list rings any bells for you.

I eat or don't eat because of:

- Stress
- Boredom
- Numbing out
- Comfort

- Escape
- Reward
- Punishment
- Bullying
- Judgment
- To look more attractive
- To maintain a certain weight or look
- Family interactions
- Work expectations
- Partner/Friend-group expectations

Are there any other examples that come up for you? Add them to your list.

Pick one of the root causes from your list and run through this practice. Then go back and pick up any others you feel describe your former relationship with food. We're getting freer and freer by the moment.

All of the reasons I use food to X (Call out one of your reasons here), I transmute and clear them.

All of the reasons X took root in me and stuck, I transmute and clear them.

All of the places I learned it, I transmute and clear them.

All of the people I associate it with and/or learned this behavior from, I transmute and clear them (again, their role, not them).

All of the reasons I haven't been able to change it if I tried, I transmute and clear them.

All of my beliefs that X is bad or shameful, I transmute and clear them.

All of my beliefs that X is necessary or absolute, I transmute and clear them.

All of my beliefs about myself tied up into X, I transmute and clear them.

All of the reasons I can't forgive myself for needing to do X, I transmute and clear them.

All of the reasons I'm afraid to change X, I transmute and clear them. All of my fear that I won't know how to replace X or what to do without it, I transmute and clear it.

With each practice, you're strengthening your connection to our divine formula.

Let's keep reclaiming.

Reclaiming Practice #5:

Deleting Food-Specific Stories

I want you to think of one food you absolutely love but have feelings of guilt or
shame about—or ones you have stories
about (like that's not very good for me).

I wanted to call this the chocolate cake practice, but then I realized not everyone loves
chocolate cake. In fact, it's not on my Top
Ten list anymore. But you get the picture.

One thing about goddess eating, which
we're going to discuss shortly, is that
we don't deny ourselves a food that will
nourish us. That's why this practice is so
important. You're going to say, "How could
something like chocolate cake nourish
me?" Let's consider some other questions.
Why does it make you happy when you eat
it? Why does it give you pleasure? Why do
you savor every morsel?

There is nothing wrong with loving a food
in and of itself. We're clearing all of your
old stories, so you no longer have to be
bound by your old pattern—self-denial *or*

bingeing. Your goddess nature knows how much to eat and enjoy.

Remember how I talked about my super-love of potato chips? They were the first food that had what we'll call hoarding energy for me. My parents would bring home a gallon of potato chips fresh from the local potato chip factory, and let me tell you: they were like manna from heaven (isn't that a story?). But those chips were the first food I remember my parents hiding away. Of course I knew where they were because I was crafty that way—they were put in the cabinets under the sink in the half-bath by the garage. I used to sneak in there, pretending to go to the bathroom, and eat some, taking great pains to put the lid back on perfectly to make sure there was no evidence. I remember being afraid of getting caught. And I also remember that other bags of chips were kept on top of the refrigerator, out of reach for us kids. My dad would binge on them after dinner. Eureka! I didn't remember that part of the story until just now—that my dad was allowed to binge on chips but we weren't—and now I can clear it.

Your associations with your "chocolate cake" food—perhaps your go-to for comfort or the focus of your denial—don't have to carry forward either. You can be free of your stories about it now, or maybe it's going to take some remembering, like it did for me, for all the details to emerge. Let it evolve. There's no timetable fixed to your goddess transformation.

If you have more than one food that fits the description, no worries. Make a list and clear them one at a time.

All right, let's bring back our goddess vision about this food(s) of yours.

Repeat after me:

All of the stories I have about this food, I transmute, clear, and delete them.

All of the emotions I have other than love and joy for X (call out your "chocolate cake" food), I transmute, clear, and delete them.

All of the ways I love this food and yet hate it at the same time, I transmute, clear, and delete them.

Everywhere X is linked to other people's stories and feelings, I transmute, clear, and delete it.

I forgive myself for believing there is anything wrong with me eating this food.

I forgive myself for believing I can't eat it as a goddess woman.

All right, now I want you to think of a food you absolutely hate. Why? Because your dislike of it might be another story. This happened to me with tomatoes. I hated them growing up, but I cleared that belief like I was guided to and discovered I love them now. Now, I'd let that story about tomatoes stand for some twenty years before clearing it.

Heck, this food might even be associated with a troubling event in your life—whether you're consciously aware of it or not—and if you clear it, you might actually like it. I remember one friend who realized they didn't like something because their mom did, and another who started hating pizza when their parents got divorced because that was the meal they'd always eaten together on family night.

Why does it matter? You don't have to do any of this—it's always your choice—but our purpose is to wipe the slate clean so we can reconnect to our divine formula. This exercise allows for the possibility of you being open to this food on your goddess menu. Heck, you may *still* not like it, but at least you've made sure it's a real dislike and not one from a story.

Ready to give it a go? Let your goddess nature show you what the food is and trust her selection. Let's clear this one (or the few that come to mind).

All of the reasons I hate this food, I transmute, clear, and delete them.

Every story I have with this food, I transmute, clear, and delete it.

Everywhere I picked this hate up from someone else or others, I transmute, clear, and delete it.

I am willing to see this food with my new goddess woman vision.

I am open to it being on my goddess menu if my goddess nature encourages it.

Using Energy to Change a Food Story

In *Goddesses Don't Do Drama,* I discussed certain relationship strategies I termed "energetic." Well, "energetic" strategies can also be used to alter our relationship with certain foods. As I said in that guide, this talk of energy might be a little woo-woo for some of you, and if it's not your cup of tea that's totally cool. You can skip ahead if you're guided to do so. But here's the thing. These strategies have worked for me and others, and I just can't refrain from sharing what I experienced around clearing my (non-life-threatening) food allergies.

I've had some interesting personal experiences with the power of woo-woo stuff, which has opened my mind to what I'll call infinite possibility. I was healed from a life-threatening illness in my mid-twenties, and I've worked with healers and people in Eastern medicine to heal other chronic and physical problems, ones my doctors had concluded they just couldn't explain. Then I got the gift of healing others (energetically) myself one fine day. Sure, that's my story, but it has sprung from my goddess nature getting stronger in me and helping me become who I came here to be. This is all to say that I have an open mind when it comes to the power to change something in our bodies that isn't healthy or what I'll call optimal (what a healthy body experiences).

That includes food intolerances.

Now, I'm not making any medical claims here. I'm certainly not telling you to clear your story around going into anaphylactic shock from peanuts and then go eat a bunch. If your allergy is life-threatening, there are professionals who can help you (doctors, nutritionists, herbalists, acupuncturists, energy healers). But if you have a mild intolerance that's plagued you like I had around dairy, you might tune into your goddess nature and see if this is something you feel you want to change. You're taking full responsibility here; you're pledging to work with her to elicit this change.

Here's the story about my former dairy allergy: for years, I stayed away from milk, really creamy cheeses, and the like. Every one of my siblings had this allergy, including my mom, so it was a belief highly reinforced by the family. But when I think back, I remember one of my brothers being able to drink chocolate milk, something he'd discovered he loved at a friend's house; except my mom thought it was an aberration when it didn't affect him. Hmm...

Then one of my early spiritual teachers told me I could clear this allergy if I wanted to. At first I didn't believe her either, but since I'd experienced other supposedly impossible changes with my body, I thought, "Why not try? I could be surprised."

It took a while for me to uncover some of the stories associated with it, but I'm not allergic to milk anymore. I even drink a cappuccino every morning after decades of drinking tea. It's awesome. I'm still working on a family-inherited intolerance to onions that goes back generations, but I know I'll get there. I just keep clearing those stories and testing the waters by eating food with a little onions in it, gauging how my body is reacting.

Interested in seeing what might happen to you? Repeat after me:

All of the reasons I have an intolerance to X (call out the food here), I transmute, clear, and delete them.

All of the times I was told I have an intolerance to X, I transmute, clear, and delete them.

All of the people involved in these stories, I transmute, clear, and delete them.

All of the stories about it being genetic, I transmute, clear, and delete them.

All of the root causes to this intolerance, I transmute, clear, and delete them.

I forgive myself for believing I'm intolerant to X.

I allow my body to come into perfect alignment with X once again.

I am willing to let it nourish me.

Does all this sound impossible? That's what I used to say. One thing about living like a goddess woman is being open to claiming and doing the impossible.

Reclaiming Practice #6:
Clearing Out the Media Blitz

Like I said, we are blitzed with stories about food in the media, anything from what we shouldn't eat (with tantalizing pictures, no less) to what's supposedly healthy for us. It's exhausting, isn't it? How about we wipe the slate clean here too?

Repeat after me:

All of the stories I've picked up about food and eating from the media, I transmute, clear, and delete them.

All of the ways my eating habits have been (or are) informed by the media, I transmute, clear, and delete them.

All of the feelings these commercials, billboards, cooking shows, or news programs foster in me, I transmute, clear, and delete them.

All of the cravings or urges I have for food that stem from the media and not my goddess woman self, I transmute, clear, and delete them.

Everywhere I'm buying into their stories and not listening to my goddess nature, I transmute, clear, and delete it.

Everywhere I think they know better than me, I transmute, clear, and delete it.

All of the power I've given them over eating and food—either consciously or unconsciously— I transmute, clear, and delete it.

Everywhere I am choosing foods because "they" tell me to, I transmute, clear, and delete it.

Yay, you, goddess woman. Take a breath. This is terrific work. How about this?

I am a goddess woman, and my choices are my own. Always.

You're taking more of your power back around eating in your life.

RECLAIMING PRACTICE #7:

Letting Go of the Number(s)

If you've ever counted calories, tried to maintain a certain weight or dress size, lose a certain number of pounds, calculated your body mass index, etc.—basically linked eating to a number—then this is the practice for you.

Numbers can be helpful, but when they start driving our decisions over our goddess woman nature and making us feel shame or anger, you are trapping your goddess woman self in a cage.

You are not a number.

Your self-image is not defined by a number. Your food choices aren't defined by a number.

Are you ready to believe that?

Your goddess nature is going to show you how (or if) you want to dance with these numbers from now on. One thing I've discovered is that I don't feel the need to weigh myself anymore. I can tell when my pants aren't fitting as well or when things are a little heavier around the waist. I don't step on the scale before or after I work out, for example, to see if there was the slightest change. I don't obsess about it. I get weighed if I go for a physical, but nothing more. That's what my goddess nature has guided me to do.

Now you get to decide how this is going to look for you. To free ourselves completely, we're going to do some more clearing.

Repeat after me:

All of the numbers I have going on in my head about eating and my body, I transmute, clear, and delete them.

All of the numbers about my weight, calories, body mass, nutritional facts, saturated fats, cholesterol, etc., I transmute, clear, and delete them.

Everywhere food is associated with numbers in my mind, I transmute, clear, and delete it.

All of the reasons it got like this, I transmute, clear, and delete them.

All of the reasons I let it get like this, I transmute, clear, and delete them.

All of the power I've given these numbers, I transmute, clear, and delete it.

Everywhere I feel bad or limited by these numbers, I transmute, clear, and delete it.

All of the people and places I learned this from, I transmute, clear, and delete them.

All of the reasons I feel trapped by the numbers, I transmute, clear, and delete them.

All of the reasons I think they will help me, I transmute, clear, and delete them.

All of the pressure I put on myself to meet certain guidelines, I transmute, clear, and delete it.

All of the pressure people put on me about them, I transmute, clear, and delete it.

I allow myself to let all these numbers go right now.

I allow myself to stop striving so hard to make them all work for me.

I allow my goddess nature to show me a happier and easier way.

I love myself enough to choose this new way.

I have the power to choose the best way for me.

Whew! Did it feel like all of those numbers were floating out of your brain? That's how it felt for me. There were a lot of them too—ones you might not have even realized were clogging up your goddess mind.

This feels so much better, so much freer.

Perhaps you're wondering what happens next, after we clear out all of this junk.

You're ready for goddess eating.

And since I can hear some of you groaning because this is too close to mindful eating or conscious eating or all of the other stuff you might have come across on this topic, let's clear that quickly too before we talk about your goddess menu.

RECLAIMING PRACTICE #8:

Blasting Out the Cynicism

You know what to do, so let's not dilly-dally. Repeat after me:

All of the stories I carry that I've heard it all before, tried it all before, and nothing ever changes for me, I transmute and clear them.

All of the reasons I'm so tired of this crap, I transmute and clear them.

All of the places where I store these negative triggers, prejudices, and cynicism, I transmute and clear them.

All of the reasons I don't want to let my new relationship with food to begin, I transmute and clear them.

Everywhere I don't feel like I can do it, I transmute and clear it.

Everywhere I'm convinced I'll never be a full goddess woman outright, especially when it comes to food, I transmute and clear it.

All of the reasons I'm certain I'm going to fail, I transmute and clear them.

Our egos can be tough customers, especially when we delve beyond our typical comfort zones. But we don't listen to them anymore. We listen to our inner goddess women rather than the hurt and shame-filled whispers of our egos.

Remember how we've talked about how our relationship with food is really about our relationship with ourselves? Yeah. This part of you—the part that felt (or feels) like she'll never measure up; the part that was told perhaps over and over by someone she loved that she would *never* be good enough—needs some love and cherishing too. And she needs a good injection of goddess faith. Feeding our emotional needs may help silence that upset ego-charged voice for a while; certainly, it should soften it.

This isn't all on your shoulders, thankfully. Your goddess nature will guide you, and she and the Universe are waiting to see if you want their help. All you have to do is hold out your hand.

Are you holding it out?

Because it's time to get started on your new goddess-tailored partnership with food.

What do you want on your menu?

CHAPTER 6

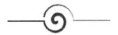

Goddess Eating: Part 1

Since we believe in the absolute perfection of our goddess bodies and we're starting to trust ourselves again when it comes to food, we're going to take it a step further. We're going to listen to what our bodies want/ask for when it comes to food.

But, Ava, you might be saying. I do listen to it, and all I do is eat that extra cupcake or popcorn at the movies. Look where it's gotten me.

This is where we need to distinguish between what our goddess woman self is saying/urging (the kind, encouraging voice) and our ego (the one who has all the stories). The same voice that urges you to be skeptical of any discussion of goddess eating may also be dispensing advice that is not beneficial to you. But this is not just about listening.

Because a goddess woman loves herself, she also makes informed decisions for herself about her life. She takes responsibility for those choices, and she holds herself accountable for them. That includes food and eating. We're talking big-time goddess shoes here (I'm putting on some silver sparkle pumps). Are you ready to step back into yours?

But first of all, I feel like I need to make a few statements about this section:

- I am not going to tell you what to eat.
- I am not going to tell you how to eat it or how to chew it, etc.
- I am not going to tell you when to eat it.
- I am not going to tell you how much or how little to eat.

Why did I feel the need to say all this? Because there is SO MUCH out there already like this—and many of you aren't feeling very empowered by it. Who can blame you? Many of you grew up with people telling you what to eat, how to eat, when to eat, or what not to eat. And there are plenty of books out there on things like nutrition, the healing properties of food, and the like, ones I've benefitted from, especially early on in my goddess transformation (I'll include a few resources at the back if your goddess self points you in that direction).

But that's not how we're going to do it here. **You're a goddess woman.** This whole journey in *The Goddess Guides* is about you living a life on your own terms based on *your* choices, with love and joy at its core. Because that's who you truly are.

Why would eating be any different?

Besides, there are some things I've observed in the world about eating, health, and weight that have led me to believe our relationship with food really *is* heavily influenced by our stories around it.

The extensive travel I've done has helped me see some pretty interesting phenomena when it comes to food. I go to Paris and see people eating *baguette* daily and foods with butter-drenched sauces and staying thin; sure, they walk everywhere, but is that the only reason? I haven't observed a lot of Parisians denying themselves food. In fact, food is part of the French formula, *joie de vivre*, which in my personal opinion is a *divine* formula at its core.

And what about the prevalence of pasta in Italy, where olive oil is also a staple of every meal? There's probably something else going on here too, but one thing I know from having worked as an apprentice chef in a northern Italian restaurant is that Italians don't eat pasta as an entrée like Americans do; and, like the French, they consider food its own art form, something to be both honored and celebrated, usually with friends and family.

Now, I was raised to "believe" (pay attention to that word) that overloading on carbs was bad for you and made you fat. That doesn't seem to be the case for many of the people I encountered in my travels. I could go on...

Sure, there are a lot of factors at work here besides food, including amount of physical activity, serving size, body chemistry, natural ingredients, etc., but the fact is: people eat different foods all the time in different parts of the world with different outcomes. It's why nutritionists want to pull their hair out sometimes. They can't easily explain why people, say in Paris, are still healthy according to the tests (we're back to numbers here, folks) they use and aren't experiencing obesity like other people who favor so-called butter- or fat-rich foods.

I couldn't possibly tell you what to eat and when, because you're the expert on you, not me: your goddess woman self knows what nourishes you and gives you joy. That's why *you're* going to decide what works best for you in the end. It's your life. Your body is your gift, and it's your responsibility. You're going to know what feels good to you—and if you remember anything, remember this: the happiness we're looking for is sustained happiness or joy, not the fleeting kind that you might have experienced briefly in one of your old moments of bingeing or starving, or when you liked the number you saw on the scale.

If you don't know what sustained happiness or joy really feels like, you might have to clear any stories that stand in the way of you experiencing it when it comes to what you eat. Maybe you'll feel guided to experiment with new things to eat or new ways of eating. It's something your goddess woman self gets to dance with as you decide what's on your Goddess Menu. And it's probably going to change throughout your life, just like a menu at a good restaurant updates its options. You'll flow with those changes and keep on nourishing yourself.

Nourishing yourself is the constant.

So let's talk turkey (pun intended) about what goddess eating looks like.

BEING IN TUNE WITH YOUR GODDESS WOMAN BODY

When you live your life as a goddess woman, you are connected to your true nature. Your wiring to our divine formula has been reestablished. You see food as nourishing, and you clear any stories that come up about food or your interaction with it that aren't. All of that means you're going to make goddess-centered choices about food for yourself.

As we've discussed, the relationship with

your goddess self is a partnership. Let's remember. She's the kind, gentle, and encouraging voice who helps you remember who you truly are. And that naturally translates to your relationship with food being a partnership. How will this affect your day-to-day life? As a goddess woman, you're going to start shopping at the grocery store differently. You're going to pay attention to the food products your goddess gaze settles on. Maybe you'll notice you've come across X product for the third time that week and finally realize your goddess self has been trying to get your attention and wants you to buy it.

This is going to be true for those of you who have a life partner or hubby as well as kids. You're going to start asking your goddess self what they need too, especially when the kids are little and you're preparing their meals. But I also encourage you to ask them for their input...because sometimes their choices will be spot on if they are still super connected to their divine nature. Sure, they might go gaga about candy because they have stories influencing them too, but you might be surprised here.

How about an example? One day a couple of years ago, I came across a food in the grocery store that I'd never tried before: goji berries. I felt I needed them. My eyes found them on the shelf, and I just had this urging. I didn't know anything about them, but my goddess nature had my attention. I bought them. Easy peasy.

When I got home, I looked them up online because I wanted to know more about them; I suppose I could have done this in the store too, but I trusted my intuition enough to just buy them in the moment. It turned out they are really great for adrenal fatigue, I discovered, among other things. I was like, aha! I was emotionally overtaxed and stressed from the death of my thirty-nine-year-old best friend, a move to a new state, and two close friends' divorces.

Over the course of my grief and supporting my other friends through their life changes, I consumed goji berries in my tea nonstop. Then one day—when my grief was mostly past and things in my life were more set-tled—I stopped consuming them. I didn't want them anymore. My body didn't need them anymore.

Some of you might be groaning, thinking this new food partnership only extends to healthy food. Goji berries, right? But what if it's something like a really beautiful rib eye steak? You might rejoice at that prospect. I love steak, and it makes me happy when I eat it. Sometimes I need the iron— something I can feel in my body, especially around my menstrual cycle (some of you who've studied nutrition may be thinking I need zinc, but it's mostly iron for me).

But other food nudges are about my goddess nature pointing out a really great food item, maybe one that's super fresh and delicious. The other day I was talking to the butcher I love at the store, and my gaze landed on the tuna in the case. I usually am not drawn to fish as a dinner choice, but this time I could feel a sense of excitement. I asked my butcher about it, and he said the tuna had just arrived and was absolutely incredible. I bought some straight away, and he was right. It was fresh and tender and delicious. I was glad I'd listened to the nudge and stepped outside of my normal choices.

Other times, my goddess nature has suggested I eat something I love, like cheddar cheese or olives or passion fruit sorbet. In those cases, I know she's helping me be present to one simple, life-changing truth about our divine formula. Eating can become a celebration. I'm eating what I love, and since nourishment is about cherishing, I'm cherishing myself and celebrating our divine formula. I am not just eating another meal because I need to eat for sustenance.

Your goddess woman self will draw you to buy food that will make you happy, yes (just as we discussed about shopping in *Goddesses Are Sexy*), but also food that's in alignment with what your body needs. Do I always eat steak? No. But once I started to listen to what my body wanted, I realized I eat it more in colder months and closer to my period.

I started to pay attention, and I keep listening. Daily.

The problem most of us have in our early experiences with Goddess Eating is that we've been listening to other voices for a long time—the ego, who thinks we should make healthy choices (remember all that dieting junk?) but doesn't really want to eat that chicken breast because it's so-called lean, or that bowl of strawberries because it's healthy, or that cup of yogurt because it's supposed to be low-fat and good for our gut. It doesn't matter if we think it's healthy if we don't want to eat it. That's still not goddess eating. This is why we need to wipe the slate clean—to erase these loaded stories so we can want to eat things again—like we did to the stories we thought we weren't partial to.

Our goddess instincts have been covered up by layers and layers of stories, so they're likely new to you. If you shower your goddess woman self with attention, listening to her enough to recognize her voice, she'll be your best friend again. Of course, it'll take some time to get there. Remember how I talked about our goddess transformation being a process?

But here's where your goddess nature helps you...

When you have an urge or an instinct to eat something, you're going to ask yourself:

Where is this coming from?

Here's a good way of sussing out if the urge is a relic of your former relationship with food. You remember how we went through the stories that helped root you to your old outlook? Think of those stories as an old boyfriend who emails or texts you out of the blue. You're not with him anymore and the reasons you broke up are still solid, but you feel a tug back in that direction, toward the past, because of the unexpectedness of the message. If you're not sure where the instinct to eat has come from, consider whether this might have happened to you. If so, no worries! There's no harm so long as you recognize the tug for what it is. It's emotion coupled with an old story you have not yet fully cleared. Or maybe it was triggered by a visit from a star in one of your old stories; can we say your mother? Or pick a person.

This is *not* your goddess woman nature urging you onward!

She wouldn't say anything to shame you. Okay, sometimes she might lovingly point out where you're not being true to yourself, which might piss you off for a second. But you're getting pissed really at yourself, aren't you? Because you know what was a goddess urge and what wasn't.

Looking for other guideposts? You can ask yourself other questions about your food inclinations until you're completely certain where the urge to eat X originates. Here are some examples:

- Am I comforting or punishing myself by eating X?
- Have I used this food as a go-to before in my old stories?
- Does my goddess woman self feel a need for love or acceptance or forgiveness about something going on in my life?
- Am I in the grip of shame about myself and my body?
- Am I feeling completely out of control or starved?

The key here is to agree to be completely honest with yourself (no blind spots).

By asking these simple questions (and any others your goddess nature helps you ask), you're going to know if this food choice is a Goddess Decision—something we talk about a lot more in *Goddesses Decide*. The more you practice listening to your goddess nature in all things, the easier it becomes.

Many of you have learned a little about my BFF from other guides, but she's a great example of the process I'm talking about. After she fully committed to being a goddess woman every day, she'd text me this one phrase a lot: *Listening is hard. Does this get any easier?*

I remembered feeling the same way when it was new to me, but it did get easier. And pretty quickly. For my BFF, it took her about a month to be done with the story that listening to her goddess nature was hard. Now it's second nature to her.

With your commitment and daily practice, it will become second nature to you too. Know why? You've restored your direct connection to your goddess woman self—the one that got trampled on by all the stories you'd picked up. Now, you just have to start paying attention to the regular signals going through the cables, and communication goes both ways. You ask her, and she answers. She lovingly suggests something, and you listen and follow through.

I think it's time for some goddess woman stories so we can see how this whole Goddess Eating thing plays out.

Jessica was cramming hard for a midterm, and she had to force herself to eat. The school library didn't allow food inside, and it was inconvenient to pack up her school books from the prime spot she'd snagged. But she'd learned the importance of feeding her brain, and she was asking it to absorb all of the dates and places and events for her history exam. How was it supposed to do that without any fuel?

The week leading up to her Friday class, she found herself craving guacamole when she'd pass by the Mexican restaurant on the way to her college. She finally gave in on the second day and stopped there for lunch.

Leading up to the exam, she also found herself craving butter, which wasn't typical for her. She'd load it on the muffin or bread she grabbed from the college cafeteria for breakfast.

On Thursday, she and her good friend, Sheri, met for dinner at one of the campus' nicer dining halls, which allowed them to both eat and study. Her friend had also mentioned she was starving from all the studying. Jessica made a comment about her strange urges for butter and guacamole all week even though she felt a little self-conscious about it.

Sheri only laughed. "Butter and avocados are really good for your brain, silly. I crave cheese when I'm cramming for a test. I think it's the saturated fats or something."

Jessica was glad to have her impression confirmed. She'd thought it was okay to listen to her body. It never steered her wrong, but eating butter and tons of guac had been a little out of left field.

On Friday, she didn't skip breakfast even though she was nervous. She loaded up a piece of bread with Irish butter—her favorite—and some special lavender honey her mom had stocked in her apartment. Then she took her history mid-term and felt really good about it. After she handed it in, she went home and slept for the rest of the day.

On Monday, Jessica found out she'd scored a B+ on her exam; Sheri came up to her after class and shared she'd gotten an A-.

"We should celebrate," her friend said.

They decided on the Mexican place since it was a student favorite. When they arrived, the server immediately asked if they wanted to start with chips and salsa and guacamole.

Sheri looked over at Jessica and winked. "Are we going to need two orders of guacamole? My friend here has been on a guac roll."

Jessica took a moment to consider the offer, but she wasn't hungry for it anymore. "Actually, I think I'm over that. Salsa only for me."

The server nodded, and as she left, Jessica checked in with herself to see if her butter craving had curbed too. Yep.

"I'm glad you told me about the whole brain thing, Sheri," she told her friend. "I usually listen to my body, but that butter thing was a little weird."

They both laughed and hunkered down in the red-pleather booth to celebrate their good fortune.

* * *

Susan loved going out with her husband on date night. The new Americana restaurant they were trying out that night was known for its cocktails. But when they arrived and the server handed her their drink menu, nothing sounded good.

Her husband was running his finger down all of the choices, a crooked smile of delight on his face.

"Hey," she called softly.

It took him a moment, but he peeled his gaze from the menu. "Wow. They've got some awesome combinations here. I mean, lemon-flavored kombucha with basil and bourbon? I've gotta try that. What are you getting, hon?"

"You aren't going to believe this," she said. "Nothing sounds good."

He reared back. "Seriously?"

"Yeah," she said. "Weird, huh? But I'm not going to push it. Maybe my body just doesn't want a drink tonight."

"No wine even?" he asked. "I hate to have you miss out on a treat. They have a great selection."

"It's fine," she said. "And I won't miss out."

Truth be told, Susan didn't even want to take a sip of Howie's drink when he offered it. He was a little concerned, but she laughed and ate heartily. The lamb shank was delicious, and she couldn't get enough of the parmesan-crusted Brussels sprouts.

When they went out three nights later with friends, she discovered she still didn't feel like drinking. Howie gave her a pensive glance when she ordered a club soda with lime. But one of her girlfriends leaned in and whispered, "Are you guys pregnant?"

Susan felt her mouth part. "Ah, not that I know of." But then she started racking her brain, trying to remember when she'd had her last period. When she realized she was a little late, she guessed it was possible. *Whoa!* Her head spun.

"I didn't even know you guys were trying," Judy said.

She felt a nervous laugh escape her mouth. "We aren't. We're happy with our boys." Sure, she'd love to have a little girl to go shopping with, but the sun rose and set on her two guys. She adored them.

Could she really be pregnant? She knew diaphragms sometimes failed. Could that be why she hadn't felt like drinking? Was her body trying to tell her something?

She tried to hold it together, but Howie knew something was up. When he dramatically yawned after their entrees were cleared, she knew he wanted to get her alone to talk. Sure enough, the minute they said goodbye to their friends, he turned to her.

"What's going on in that beautiful head? I've been dying to know all night."

They were always open with each other, and even though she wasn't sure if she was pregnant, she wasn't going to dance around the possibility. He was her partner.

"Judy asked me if I wasn't drinking because I was pregnant," she said.

Howie started laughing. He even slapped his knee.

But when she only gave him a smile, he stopped gradually, as if in slow motion.

"*Oh*," he said, his mouth parting like hers had earlier.

"Let's stop by the drug store on the way home," she said. "Might as well see."

Howie started jabbering about when it might have happened—something he did when he got nervous. She fisted her hands to her belly and tried to keep calm. Though another pregnancy hadn't been part of their plan, she realized she wanted this. She would love to have another baby.

When they got home, Howie paid the babysitter and saw her out. Susan was looking in on their two boys all cuddled up in their twin beds when he found her.

"Looking at them like this, all I can think of is having another," he whispered. "In case you were wondering."

She turned to him and stroked his face. "I'm glad. I would be so happy if it's true."

He took her hand. "Let's find out."

In the bathroom, he sat on the rim of the tub while she took the test and then pulled her into his arms as they read the result. Sure enough, she was pregnant. Her body had been trying to tell her something was different.

She threw her arms around him, and he spun her in a circle, both of them laughing with joy.

* * *

Leah was working a double shift at the hardware store when she started sneezing. Not once, but five times. She shook her head when the sneezing fit ended and continued stocking the shelves. When she took her break, she found herself craving grapefruit. All she wanted was a juicy, ruby red fruit covered with a little honey—the way she preferred it.

Since she was getting off late, it didn't make sense to go to the grocery store. But she was still craving grapefruit when her shift ended. She wondered if she was getting a cold. She'd been working a lot of hours and not sleeping as much, and all that sneezing that had come out of the blue.

Even though she was exhausted, she stopped by the store and picked up a bag of grapefruits. When she got home, she found herself eating not one but two. The flavor seemed to saturate her mouth, and she savored every bite. Loved having the juice run down her chin even.

In the morning, she was still hungry for grapefruit, which seemed crazy, but she listened to her body, something her mother had taught her. She had a grapefruit for breakfast, and then prepared a second one so she could have it for lunch.

She found she had more energy at work that day and decided the grapefruit had to be boosting her system. All the Vitamin C goodness.

When she looked in her fridge the next morning, trying to figure out what she wanted for breakfast, her eyes landed on the half-full bag of grapefruits. They weren't appealing anymore. She laughed. What on Earth was she going to do with all of them?

* * *

When Patty walked into the break room at work, her gaze immediately fell to the plate of cookies sitting on the table. Gena Marie was always bringing in her homemade baked goods because she loved trying new recipes, and it was really sweet and all—but it was also sometimes hard to resist.

Patty thought about it for a moment, and then decided she was going to treat herself. Eating one of Gena Marie's double chocolate chip cookies was going to brighten her day. As she sunk her teeth into the chewy morsel, she did a little dance in the kitchen.

"Somebody's happy," she heard Gena Marie say behind her.

Her mouth was full, so it took Patty a moment to finish chewing. "Did my dance give me away?" she asked.

"And the moaning," Gena Marie said, laughing, punching her lightly in the arm. "I love it when people moan over my cookies, especially the men. I keep hoping Gary is going to ask me out."

Gary worked in the finance department. "He sure is cute," Patty replied. "Thanks for baking cookies, Gena Marie. Made my day."

"And your little dance made mine," the other woman said.

As Patty left the break room, she found herself smiling. A cookie had improved both of their days. Sometimes the little things meant a lot.

Is all of this starting to make sense? As goddess women, we sometimes have to pause to listen to our goddess woman bodies and selves to see what they truly want. And it doesn't always have to be something "healthy," right? Patty decided to treat herself to a cookie and made a celebration out of it.

The biggest aspect of goddess eating is being in tune with yourself and eating from that place. We listen. We decide. We enjoy. We take responsibility for what we're eating, and we do so in a way that allows our systems to work easily. We're partners with our goddess bodies in all our choices.

How about we turn to our goddess tool so this process goes back to being automatic?

Reclaiming Practice #9:

Tuning In Goddess Style

Let's clear anything left in the way of you listening to and *trusting* your goddess woman self and your body. Maybe you still fear failure. Take a breath, goddess woman, and remember that it's a process. If you end up eating something you later regret, something your ego drove you toward, big deal. You can stop the shame in its tracks. You love yourself, and you have the power to clear whatever story you have going on about what you just did—even if you ate something you knew would make you feel sick, like a bucket full of leftover Halloween candy.

It's okay!

Food isn't your enemy. Remember that. It's only your old stories that have risen back up, trying to reroot themselves inside you. Maybe stress triggered you or a call from your sister who fat shames you. We talk a lot about surrounding yourself with people who love and support the goddess woman you are in *Goddesses Don't Do Drama,* and if you have food shamers in your life, people who cut you down because of your weight or food consumption, you might want to check out that guide for some help. No goddess woman needs to put up with that kind of cruelty and bullying—even amongst people who purport to be your family, spouse, or friends.

Now, are you ready to clear these insecurities?

Repeat after me:

Everywhere I'm still not fully connected to my goddess self or body about food yet, I transmute, clear, and delete it.

All of the old signals still working under the radar, I transmute, clear, and delete them.

All of the reasons I believe I won't be able to know what my goddess self is telling me about food, I transmute, clear, and delete them.

Everywhere I'm afraid to listen, I transmute,

clear, and delete it.

All of the changes I fear it will create in my life and me, I transmute, clear, and delete them.

All of the reasons I don't think I can do this, I transmute, clear, and delete them.

All of the reasons I still don't want to try, I transmute, clear, and delete them.

Everywhere I'm afraid I'll fail, I transmute, clear, and delete it.

USING YOUR GODDESS BRAIN TO SEE WHAT'S TRUE

Another component of goddess eating has to do with your brain. You're smart, goddess woman, in case you didn't know it. I'm not talking about book smart or street smart, though you may well be one or both.

I'm talking goddess smart.

Our brains are able to figure things out, make associations, and store information. They're masterpieces when you think about it. Being smart about the food you eat as a goddess woman is part of your partnership with your body.

For example, now that most of us buy so much of our food from manufacturers, one of the outcomes—if that's the story we want to go with—is that there are plenty of packaging gimmicks our goddess brains need to parse, telling us what's real and what's not. Pretty packaging doesn't necessarily make it a better product, let alone the right product for me. I decide that for myself.

Another piece of this is paying attention to changes to what I'm calling the natural process of foods and animals.

Let's look at an example for guidance. I don't read a lot of labels for food anymore since I'm in tune with my goddess nature, but recently one phrase seemed to jump off the package as I was looking at eggs. I love eggs—all ways, all kinds.

This package said the eggs were from vegetarian hens, and my goddess brain was like, *what?* Remember, I'm the first generation off the farm, but I was put to bed at night with farm stories when I visited my grandma. I knew chickens eat meat some-times. They're hunters and will eat a mouse or a snake in a heartbeat. But I also remem-bered horror stories of one of them get-ting hurt and the rest of them pecking it to death and eating it.

When I came home from the store, I did some research to make sure. Maybe I was even remembering it wrong.

It turns out my memory had served me well. Chickens are omnivores, but some people prefer to eat the eggs of vegetarian chickens—whether because they believe it's healthier or because they are vegetarians and feel the decision fits in better with their lifestyle. I choose to believe (my story) that these eggs aren't any more special because they came from vegetarian hens; it might be that they're actually a less nutrition-rich product because of the changes to a chick-en's normal diet. You can listen to your goddess nature's guidance and decide for yourself. That's what this is all about.

INTENTIONAL FOOD CHOICES

As we just discussed, you have an incredible

brain, goddess woman. Did you also know you can use it to find foods that can help support or boost your body or address a physical condition?

Here's another example from my own life. For over a decade, I struggled with sadness and depression, a condition that went along a string of medical issues. I used to have chronic respiratory infections, sometimes one a month for three or four months in a row. I would go to the doctor and gets meds for the bacterial infection and get better, but a couple of weeks later, the virus would surge back up again. The condition in my lungs and sinuses would intensify again, almost worse than before because my body wasn't one-hundred-percent healthy. And so the cycle went.

All of this was way before I was living in my goddess nature; at that time in my life, I was living in a world of hurt dictated by shame-coated, fear-based, sad stories about my very self and how things had turned out for me. I wasn't what you'd call a happy person then, though I tried to be grateful. Getting through every day was sometimes a challenge, and I struggled to find hope or meaning in all the suffering I was experiencing mentally, emotionally, and physically.

But I kept searching for answers, ways to help support my body. I ended up discovering that almonds reduce lung inflammation. And what's a major aspect to a respiratory infection? Inflammation. I decided it wouldn't hurt to eat a handful of almonds a day. Now, I can't medically say with any certainty that it helped. What I can say is that my intention to support my body with my mind was a Goddess Decision. And those are the decisions that spark miracles in our lives.

Sure, almonds didn't address the root causes of my sadness and depression—I had to address those as a goddess woman—but I do believe eating almonds was one act of Goddess Eating that I engaged in at the time. I was nourishing my body with food designed to help it, the body that was so keenly suffering from my beliefs and stories and all of the emotions attached.

The wonderful thing about this modern age of ours is the access to information.

There is so much information out there about the supportive or healing properties of food. Sure, it's become an industry too, but you have a goddess brain. If you want to boost or heal something, you can trust it to find the best helpers for you.

Of course, there are also a slew of medical professionals who now specialize in nutrition—bona fide nutritionists, as well as homeopaths and herbalists. That's also available if it's something your goddess nature guides you to.

Again, food is our partner. When we listen and make decisions about what kinds will most nourish our body, we are in full alignment with our goddess woman nature and this beautiful and sexy body we have.

Dancing with Goddess Eating

Some of these concepts might be new to you, but the truth is your goddess nature came here with them.

For those of you who still think this might be too much effort, let me ask you another question:

Do you really want to go back to the way things were?

Were your old patterns with food making you feel good about yourself and your body?

I struggled for years to overcome illness and injury, and when I was at what I called my lowest, I'd ask myself if I wanted to keep living like I was. The answer was always no. I wanted a better life for myself. I wanted to be healthy again. I wanted to be free of pain and depression and loneliness. So even if I couldn't see a light at the end of the tunnel, I would fix my gaze on a spot and keep moving forward in my so-called darkness.

For those of you who have had a lifelong personal struggle with food, one you've carried for a long, long time, this might be the decision you're called upon to make.

Loving yourself and choosing to live a new way will take time. You know how it's said most habits take about three weeks to break so we can start a new normal? First, we can clear the story that it takes X days, since we're all different. And the wattage we put behind our choice can make it shorter. Know any smokers who quit cold turkey? That's pure will, folks. Loads of it.

And will is your goddess friend—just like your intuition is.

These ideas about Goddess Eating are all for you to dance with because you're going to be eating for the rest of your life.

CHAPTER 7

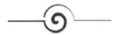

GODDESS EATING: PART 2

We've talked a lot about the food part of goddess eating and choosing foods that nourish our goddess woman bodies. But food is bigger than one meal. Eating and cooking can open us to a wider world.

Part of goddess eating is finding a new way to harness this potential and make food a positive force in your life.

Let's talk about a few of these forces, ones you might be dancing with already or ones that you hadn't thought about before.

EATING AS CONNECTION

Connection with others

When we eat from a place of divine partnership, we are connecting to our goddess woman nature. Eating is going to produce a new byproduct: joy. Why? Because when we're nourishing ourselves, we're saying this to our goddess woman self:

Hey! I love you enough to feed you and nourish this kickass body we have.

Since most of us eat more than once a day, we often eat with others. People have been cooking and eating together since forever, like we've discussed, but the goddess way is about connecting to others. And when we choose to be a goddess woman, we choose to be around other people who are also living their truth. We say no to friends or family who continually shame us about food, eating, and body image.

Being our true goddess woman selves opens us up to a whole new circle. We might find true love, that BFF we've always wanted, or a new person we feel is like a sister or brother. The sky is the limit.

We pick and choose our goddess invitations, so we actually like all the people around the dinner table. We're not there because we feel we can't say no. And we won't find ourselves sitting around the table with people who completely ignore each other, and the meal, in favor of their cell phones (something I've seen more times than I can count!).

The people you choose to dine with also won't look crossways at you if you've decided you want to eat French fries with your burger instead of a salad or make a snide comment about how you should probably not have an appetizer because you don't need to eat that much.

Being loved, seen, and heard by others is its own act of nourishment. When you bridge it with your new partnership with food, you have an endless road of joy ahead of you. The daily event of eating becomes another incredible opportunity to connect with and have fun with those you care about and love.

Maybe you and your new and old connections can even start cooking together if you like to cook. Or the one who doesn't like to cook can cut up vegetables or prep other parts of the meal for the one who does enjoy it. In my life, that's often the case. You might even pour a nice glass of wine and drink it as you cook instead of waiting to serve it with the meal. That's another European trick I learned. Why wait to enjoy your meal when the fun can start right now?

Remember. Food is life, and life is celebration. This is your time, goddess woman. Savor every minute.

Even if we find ourselves eating alone, we can still enjoy the meal. We just have to clear some stories about cooking for one, eating alone, not liking to eat at a restaurant alone, etc. Think about eating (and cooking if you like that) as a way of loving yourself and nourishing your beautiful, sexy body.

Living as a goddess woman, we don't need anyone to make us feel happy or nourished. That's ours to do. Other people are the icing on our proverbial goddess cake.

Connection to loved ones past

We human beings are an interesting lot. Our power of connection to others is so great in us that we can miss or fondly remember someone who is long since past.

For me, few things do that quite like food. I often remember my grandmother when I'm cooking since she taught me. But it's more than that. Cooking with her was usually loving and happy. From the time I could help her, I felt the love gracing her kitchen. Her recipe box was packed with special treats written from women in the family who had passed away but whose memory she still kept alive. She'd tell me stories about my great-grandmother, who had "the touch" and could always make mouth-watering—and filling—meals for her family of twelve.

I loved to see all of these women's handwriting on the recipe cards we'd pull out for a meal. Auntie Anna was legendary for her strudel recipe; she even had a drop table she would stretch the dough on. I still haven't mastered that recipe, but I smile when I think about her and that special table in the parlor she'd convert for her magical food alchemy.

Recipes take on a new meaning when they're passed down this way. We remember the deceased loved one who gave us this recipe. We smile when we share it with other people. We get to share a story about, say, our grandma, who used to make this cake or that cookie every Christmas Eve or that birthday.

Cooking connects us to love, and it can connect us to a relationship we used to enjoy.

Maybe you don't have any stories like these. Perhaps no one in your family cooked. No one kept any recipes, or they all got lost. Or you might never have liked your guardians' food in the first place. However it goes. That's okay. Maybe it's not even something that you want in your goddess woman life.

But let me leave you with this thought...

What if *you* were the one people told stories about, the one who brought back the notion of food as nourishment and stopped the old family stories of starvation or excess?

What if your children told their children how you were the one who brought back the joy for eating and guided them to live as goddess women once again?

Now *that* would be a legacy.

Connection with our culture or other cultures

Food is one of the greatest travelers on this planet. Think about how far that first pasta recipe traveled when Marco Polo brought it back from Kublai Khan's court. Or how far cinnamon traveled to London from what was then Ceylon.

It's like we've been connecting to other cultures on this beautiful planet of ours since the first food bartering, probably with the Phoenicians way back in 6000 B.C.

This might not resonate with you, and that's okay. But here's how I look at it. A dish of food has a story, and that very meal you're consuming has nourished other people, families, and sometimes even a whole culture. Sometimes it even helped it survive. Think of rice, wheat, beans, corn, cassava, and potatoes.

I've had friends who used to pick a country and cook dishes that nation was known for as a way of connecting to other cultures.

Sometimes different cuisines are blended

together to create something new and beautiful, what we call fusion in the gourmet circles. It's been going on forever. I remember eating at one of my favorite restaurants in the world—in a beautiful old Roman seaside village outside of Beirut— where they combined very typical Lebanese food with Spanish cuisine. The result was breathtaking.

As I nourish my goddess woman body, I love being surprised by these magical food encounters with other god men or goddess women who understand food is life.

Across the world, certain special foods are offered up to the gods, either on a daily basis or for certain rituals or celebrations (and in some cases goddesses, depending on the tradition). The Philippines even has a recipe called Food for the Gods that is a dessert-like bar made of dates. How many cultures past and present still make food offerings to their gods? What are we to glean from that?

Our takeaway is that we, as goddess women, deserve to honor our bodies with the food that will nourish us. Every day we make a nourishing offering to ourselves when we eat.

Ultimately, it's up to us to decide, but choosing to be a goddess woman and live like one means eating like one.

On our own terms.

EATING AS PRIVILEGE

The truth is, it's a privilege to be able to eat and not everyone has enough food to sustain them, something we can recognize when we open our minds and hearts.

As someone who's worked with the United Nations and other development agencies, I find it interesting that even the World Health Organization uses the word *undernourishment* when it discusses people experiencing extreme hunger. Current estimates from 2014-2016 are that 795 million people of the 7.3 billion people in the world are experiencing this serious issue.

Think about that.

I'm not bringing this up as a way to encourage you clean your plate, like when you were a kid and your parents told you shame-based stories about starving kids in Africa.

I'm only noting this because when we're all goddess women and god men—regardless of our circumstances—it might just happen that you find yourself called to compassion for another person and perhaps help them.

I used to feel unsafe around homeless men on the streets in Washington, D.C., for example. But I had friends who would offer to buy them lunch or dinner from time to time if their goddess or god selves guided them to. I've had others give their take-away bag to someone. It made an impression on me. They were doing their part to help another goddess woman or god man be nourished by food when times were tough. The same went for the food drives at school or church.

It's the moments when we realize another goddess woman or god man doesn't have enough to eat that we understand eating is also a privilege. It should be a human right, but that's a geo-political discussion and doesn't help us here.

No surprise, I used to experience this issue all the time, working in warzones. But honestly my first exposure happened much earlier—when I was working as a student volunteer on the Texas-Mexico border with kids for a summer program. It was the first time I'd ever seen real poverty, the kind where a family could only send one child per day because the kids had to share a pair of shoes; now I wonder why shoes were required at the camp. I also remember talking to my younger sister, who also volunteered, after we learned the women in the village had been saving for months to serve us chicken with mole sauce. They could only afford one chicken, you see.

Eating that meal was a privilege, let me tell you.

I made sure to thank every goddess woman involved for the meal. This was their way of thanking us for sharing our gifts with their children, who had taught me as much as I supposedly taught them.

It was the first time I was an honored guest at a meal.

But I also remember sitting in the parking lot of a major grocery chain after spending time in a country rife with famine and hunger. Usually I'd be up early from jet lag and no one else would be there. The grocery store would loom large in front of me, and I'd think of all the food standing right before me in one place and how scarce basic staples were in the place I'd come from; how expensive they were because of war and maybe corruption or hefty government taxes on importation. I had to work for years to clear the guilt I felt in those moments, but there's one lesson I've never forgotten: eating isn't something everyone is nourished by.

It just goes to show that there are other breakdowns in our divine formula:

Goddess+Food=Nourishment

Those problems are sometimes systemic, caused by war or economics or natural disasters or weather patterns such as drought.

But it doesn't make the divine formula any less true.

So, as we remember what other god men and goddess women are going through when it comes to hunger, we can be more open to what our goddess self has in store for us.

Hopefully, as you're starting to see, food isn't always just about a meal.

Let's turn to the next aspect of goddess eating.

EATING AS BLESSING

Gratitude is a goddess woman trait; how could we not be grateful for the very food that nourishes our body?

I'm not trying to say you need to bow your head before every meal or say a prayer. That's for you to decide.

But there is something special that happens when we approach our food with a blessing. I've taken to blessing where my food comes from—and who was involved in the process—because I am grateful to everyone and everything involved in bringing nourishment to my body.

Now, I was raised to say a blessing before every meal, and sometimes it felt rote and seemed like just one more thing we had to do.

As I grew up and remembered I was a goddess woman, I danced with how I wanted to bless my food and be grateful for it. I frequently send notes back to the chefs at a restaurant to thank them for sharing their gifts with me through their magical food. Who knows? That might be something that appeals to you. I've discovered how joyful it makes a person to feel appreciated.

I also remember shocking a friend when we were on a car trip by blessing my fast food with the intention that it nourish my body. He was just coming out of a time as a vegetarian and really into eating organic, locally sourced foods. That's great. But he had a story around all fast food being bad. It hadn't dawned on him that a goddess woman could bless it and ask it to nourish her body.

He hadn't believed it *could* nourish someone's body despite the fact that it was food.

Our conversations about food continued since we often cooked and ate together as friends. On a day when we shopped at the grocery store together in preparation for our meal, he expressed worry and some frustration that not all our vegetables were organic. I was like, "Don't worry. We'll just bless them so they nourish you like you think they're supposed to."

This might be sounding a little woo-woo to you, and that's okay. But the fact is, I didn't have the same story around using all organic food that he did. I wasn't feeling bad about our groceries. In fact, I was super excited about cooking and eating the meal.

Again, this is a dance, but blessing something or someone is one of the most powerful transformational acts I've discovered we can utilize as goddess women. There's no accident that the act of blessing something is folded into so many sacred religious practices.

Think of all of the blessings around food: the Catholics' practice of transubstantiation that transforms bread into the very body of Jesus Christ; certain Native American tribes' corn and buffalo dances; the Jewish celebration of Passover and the whole practice of kosher foods; the monthly observation of Ramadan and the practice of halal meats in Islam; the harvest festival of Pongal. I could keep going on. This is all to say that blessing food isn't new.

For me, in blessing food, my purpose is for it to serve my highest intention—and that's to nourish my body.

My mom actually added something a while back I now think is pretty interesting. She says, "Bless this food to the nourishment of our body, not to the fat of our bodies." That's her goddess woman intention.

Like I say in *Goddesses Decide*, goddess women have the power to ask for anything. And since we live from our goddess selves, we're always asking for things that bring about more love and joy and abundance in our lives. And since the Universe is all about that, it rises to meet our intention.

Yeah, that's how powerful you are.

CHAPTER 8

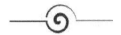

FINAL THOUGHTS:
GODDESS WOMAN FEASTING

A few years ago, I had this interesting notion that changed my whole life. I realized I wanted to feel about life like I did (even then) about food. I wanted to look forward to it. I wanted to savor it. I wanted to luxuriate in it.

Back then I wasn't as excited about life. This thought occurred in the early days of my goddess transformation when I first started clearing my old stories and letting go of all the pent-up hurt, anger, and shame I had about myself and aspects of my life experience.

I realized I wanted to feast.

Like a goddess woman.

Well, this idea coincided with another decision. One day I realized I didn't want to save the champagne in the refrigerator for a special occasion. Every day was a day to celebrate. Somehow, against so many odds, I was still alive and kicking and getting healthier and happier by the day.

My life was something to celebrate.

I was something to celebrate.

From then on, I slowly began to create moments to feast. It didn't have to involve tons of food. Some of my favorite moments were walking up to a special cheese shop in my old neighborhood when I took a break from writing midday. I'd come home and make a plate of saucisson, cheese, and maybe slice up an apple or avocado. Then I'd take a single-serving bottle of champagne and pop it or pour a glass of wine and sit at my dining room table or in my garden.

I did this all by myself. And it was so happy. It was my own personal goddess feast.

For a time, I gave up holding lavish dinner

parties because I'd been ensnared in old stories about cooking for others and some accompanying toxic relationships. But with this new goddess woman perspective, I started to enjoy having people over again; not anyone I had drama with, you can be sure, but new friends who were aligning or fully aligned with their goddess woman or god man selves.

I called these get-togethers feasts too, but it wasn't anything complicated. I'd ask my goddess woman self to suggest what we might eat, and it was interesting how many times I ended up picking food items that turned out to be my companions' favorites. Listening to your goddess nature does that. I even invited them to cook with me or help cut something up as prep; I didn't need to do it all myself like I'd believed in my old stories, ones that had made cooking for people seem burdensome and unhappy.

Our feasts were community activities—a beautiful way to celebrate and connect with each other, to feel nourished even.

Sometimes we even turned on music and danced around the kitchen.

We were feasting before we even sat down at the table—goddess style.

Sound interesting? Is your goddess woman nature curious how this might look for you?

This goddess woman not only likes to feast now; she sees life as a feast—one for the senses, for the heart, for her curiosity.

And she's nourished by every part of it, including the food.

Give it a try, goddess woman.

Your life feast is just beginning.

CHAPTER 9

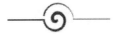

AVA'S FAVORITE FOOD-ESQUE RESOURCES

Like I said, this guide isn't meant to speak about things like nutrition or the healing properties of foods, but in case it's useful, here are a few of my favorite resources that have helped me.

Healing With Whole Foods: Asian Traditions and Modern Nutrition

By Paul Pitchford

When I was working with my body to heal from chronic pain and other issues, one of my former teachers recommended this guide to me. It's a treasure trove of information, and I've used it to help myself and those I love through various sicknesses, including the effects of long-term illnesses.

The Big Book of Juices: More Than 400 Natural Blends for Health and Vitality Every Day

By Natalie Savona

My goddess self helped me find this book when I was looking for a way to both detox my body from a buildup of medicine and heavy metals from my illnesses and surgeries as well as boost my immune system if I came down with a cold.

Nourishing Traditions: The Cookbook that Challenges Politically Correct Nutrition and the Diet Dictocrats

By Sally Fallon

I actually can't remember if my old teacher recommended this book or not, and I haven't looked at it for a while, but I was guided to include this one as well. It has a lot of interesting discussion about food and nutrition in the beginning, before she gets into the cookbook.

The Nourishing Traditions Book of Baby & Child Care

By Sally Fallon

I was also guided to share another book of Sally's for those of you who have children in case you are interested in these topics as well.

Again, these are resources I have found helpful in my own goddess eating. If they resonate with you as a goddess woman, check them out.

GENERAL TOOLS
FOR CONNECTING TO
YOUR GODDESS NATURE

While each of *The Goddess Guides* is focused on a specific topic, there are some general tools I wanted to pass along that I've found helpful for getting in touch with one's goddess nature. I'm sharing this chapter—like the introduction—in all of the guides because they bookend the highest purpose of our journey here: connecting to our goddess nature.

Since connection to ourselves is key, here are a few simple ways to reconnect to one's self.

SIMPLE HEART CONNECTORS

Place your hand over your heart. Listen for the heartbeat. Breathe. Take as long as you need to feel reconnected.

To me, it's a feeling of calm followed by the warmth of love radiating through the body. You'll feel what you feel.

You can also simply affirm to yourself: *I love and accept myself.* This affirmation is one of the most powerful ones I know, and repeating it like a mantra can change your whole energy. It's like giving yourself a hug and throwing yourself a private party for being you.

Another way of connecting to the heart involves folding your fingers into your palms and placing your knuckles together over your heart. This is called "Bear Pose," and it activates the heart chakra beautifully and connects the energies of the body.

If you have a lot of blocks in your body, it might take a while before you start to feel your own energy. I recommend working on transmuting and deleting the stories creating the blocks—like we've done around specific topics in these guides.

Hugging It Out

Out of sync with a loved one? I recommend what I call "hugging it out."

One of my best friends taught this to me, and at first, I was so uncomfortable. He'd hold me for minutes. I was aware of his body and his breath. I thought, "When is he going to let me go?" But I knew he was expressing his love for me, and I didn't want to cut him off. I also knew I needed to work on the reasons for my discomfort.

I knew being held by someone I completely loved and trusted, who loved and trusted me, shouldn't cause me discomfort. My friend was teaching me how to receive love through a hug, and not just a little "I love you" hug, but a whole body, "I'm so glad you're in my life and love you to pieces" hug.

He was also getting us in sync with each other, and I discovered very quickly that a long hug like that between two willing parties (okay, I was determined too) creates a harmony in energies.

"Hugging it out" is also the perfect antidote

to those moments or days when we aren't feeling much love and joy whatsoever. Ask someone for a hug if you need it.

Around my house, we commonly ask someone who doesn't seem like themselves, "Do you need a hug?" It's our go-to and has transformed person-to-person interactions faster than anything I've ever seen.

Energy Booster & Grounder

Looking for more energy? Who doesn't want that? Putting your hand on the crown of your head works wonders. Depending on how tired you are, you might need to leave it there for a while or even tap it to break up some of the blockages there. The energies in the body rise up to meet your hand. That's why it works. Again, the power of touch, right?

Stomping your feet also works wonders. Again, the energy you generate by stomping your feet also stirs the energies.

And it helps ground you if you're feeling what some people call "spacey" or "flighty." It makes you feel your feet, something

I cultivate on a daily basis given how my energy works.

Prayer & Meditation

When people ask me what I've done to become such a joyful person (trust me, I haven't always been), I note how much meditation and prayer boost my life.

Ever since I could speak, I've prayed. But when I added meditation to it, my spiritual practice became even richer.

To me, meditation isn't just about clearing your mind of thoughts. It's about connecting to the love in your heart, which spreads out to your whole being. That's what calms the mind and body and connects us to the divine. We've talked about this a lot.

To me, the only difference between a "great" meditation and "great" sex is semantics. I get to the same place—either with a partner or on my own.

You might be saying, "Seriously, Ava?" Mediation is as great as sex? Yep.

But I know not everyone has discovered this yet. I've had so many people tell me they have trouble meditating. They don't feel they're doing it right.

Most of the people who've told me this have tried to use meditation solely to clear their minds. From their thoughts, in case you were wondering.

But when they started getting in touch with their hearts like I suggested—even by something as simple as listening to their heartbeat—they found it much easier to meditate and even more powerful. It's that heart chakra piece we've discussed before.

For me, connecting to my goddess nature and the Universe or the Divine or whatever you want to call it (basically LOVE) is the single most beautiful gift I've ever given myself. It keeps delivering an endless fountain of joy.

And I do meditate as a practice every day, even if it's only for a few minutes.

But I also know I am connected to my goddess nature and the Divine at all times now in a way I never used to be, so I dance with the practice differently than I did in the past.

Your spiritual practices will evolve as you evolve. The trick is to remain open and flexible and not become rigid in these things we term "practices." And if you find yourself developing stories and beliefs around them or anything else, it's time to bring out the Blaster, our reclaiming practice. Speaking of which...

RECLAIMING PRACTICES: DELETING THE STORIES

Have a thought or a story or belief you don't want to have? We've talked about this a lot in the guides, but let's review it here again.

Simply say, *I transmute and delete X.* As many times as you need to blast it out. Or you can use, *I forgive myself for believing X.*

Need to forgive someone and release yourself from negative interactions in your life?

Just repeat, *X, I release you from the role you are playing for me. Go in peace. All is forgiven and released.*

Feeling pissed off?

I surround my anger with light and love; all is forgiven and released.

Not sure what your stories are? Listen to yourself. Ask the Universe to show them to you. Maybe even ask a loving friend for his or her thoughts. Or work with a professional.

Your goddess nature will help guide you. Trust me. The stories will come up when you decide to take this journey of self-discovery and healing. Your goddess nature has mandated it.

EASY CALMING PRACTICE

Need help calming yourself down from anxiety, paranoia, or hysteria?

Try saying the sound "Heeee," either to yourself or out loud.

I've had friends do this, and they suddenly felt light-headed. Why? Because they were so amped up on anxiety and worry, the corresponding relief their system experienced was tremendous. Pent-up emotion sometimes does that on its way out. It's like we've turned our emotional faucet on high, and it's flooding out of us.

But trust me... This one is a winner. I used it on many scary nights in warzones when I'd jump at every sound or simply couldn't sleep because I was too anxious to rest.

FANNING

Huh? Yeah, you heard me. Get out a magazine or a piece of paper—or even a real Spanish lace ladies' fan. When you feel sluggish or crummy, fan yourself. Why? It breaks the heavy energy up in your energetic field. And it works... I taught this to my sister to help my niece when she was super little. She was picking up a lot of junk from other kids at daycare, and fanning brushed it off. Her mood immediately improved. She was happy again and back to herself. It's funny, but when she was three years old, she started picking up a magazine and fanning her mother when she had a "bad" day at the hospital. My niece knew what to do. She was still in touch with her goddess nature.

Native Americans and other cultures have been using this practice—likely under different names—for centuries. I can't recommend it enough.

Simple Chakra Openers

Curious about opening up your chakras more after all this talk about how it opens us up to more love and joy in the body?

Here are a couple of simple ways: color and sound. You can wear a color you feel drawn to or one you intuit you need to boost your energy.

And you can say the sound of that chakra out loud or to yourself. I loved seeing that "Yum," something I say all the time for good food, was the heart sound. Made sense to me. Food makes me happy.

Chakra	Color	Sound
Root	Red	Lum
Sacral	Orange	Vum

Solar Plexua	Yellow	Rum
Heart	Green to Pink	Yum
Throat	Turquoise	Hum
Third Eye	Indigo	Om
Crown	Purple to White	(Silent-no sound)

You can check out tons of other things about chakras online if you want. There is no limit to what you can learn.

SHIFTING PAIN, BLOCKAGES & OTHER PHYSICAL ISSUES

The body is wired to communicate your emotional, mental and spiritual nature with you. Like the stars guiding a ship, the body is your guide in this journey called life. Here are some common areas of pain and blockage and their corresponding stories along with some helpful tidbits to shift them. Of course, if they are chronic, you will likely need to deal with both the physical aspects of the situation as well as the mind-body connection.

Personally, I've experienced a lot of illness and injury in my life. Sometimes I needed to use medicine and physical therapy as well as digging deeper into the root causes of the pain. When I cleared the cause, my body healed faster and completely.

Body Signal	Story	Shift
Back	Where don't you feel supported? By yourself or others?	Write them out and do the Reclaiming practice. And nurture yourself.
Shoulders	What burdens are you carrying around? Either for yourself or others?	Write them out and do the Reclaiming practice. And nurture yourself.
Neck	What thoughts are too big to realize? To heavy to carry right now?	Write them out and do the Reclaiming practice. And nurture yourself.

Knees	What childhood issues or patterns with your parents are still playing out?	Write them out and do the Reclaiming practice. And nurture yourself.
Yeast Infections	Where do you feel ashamed in your life and actions and with whom?	Write them out and do the Reclaiming practice. Say the word Lum (for the root chakra/ genital area).
Head aches	What are you obsessing about, and where don't you feel the Divine listens or supports you?	Write them out and do the Reclaiming practice. Say the word Om or be silent.
Sore Throat	What aren't you expressing?	Write them out and do the Reclaiming practice. Say the word Hum. Draw or write something.

Heart Issues	Where do you feel not loved or incapable of love?	Write them out and do the Reclaiming practice. Say the word Ha (for the physical heart) and Yum.
Liver and Gall Bladder	Where are you frustrated, enraged, or overwhelmed?	Write them out and do the Reclaiming practice. Say the word Shoo and imagine green light surrounding the organs.
Lungs and Large Intestine	What is making you sad or what are you grieving over? What can't you let go of?	Write them out and do the Reclaiming practice. Say the word Zzzz, and imagine white light surrounding the organs.
Kidneys and Bladder	What are you afraid of? What can't you hold or carry anymore in your life?	Write them out and do the Reclaiming practice. Say the word Shwoo, and imagine turquoise light surrounding the organs.

Stomach, Spleen, Pancreas	Where don't you feel nurtured? Where can't you digest life?	Write them out and do the Reclaiming practice. Say the word Who and imagine yellow light surrounding the organs.
Hands	What are you afraid to reach for? What don't you feel you can grasp?	Write them out and do the Reclaiming practice. Link your hands in prayer-style and rotate them clockwise and counter-clockwise.
Feet	Where are you afraid to move forward? Where can't you reach?	Write them out and do the Reclaiming practice. Imagine yourself walking to the places that you're scared of, the ones you really want to go to. Believe you can do it!

Eyes	What are you afraid to see? Where can't you see the highest version of you and your life?	Write them out and do the Reclaiming practice. Repeat Om to clear your vision, and rub your hands together and lay the palms over your eyes, affirming you are willing to see.
Ears	What are you afraid to hear? What can't you hear to help you receive the guidance you need?	Write them out and do the Reclaiming practice. Rub your hands together and lay the palms over your ears, affirming you are willing to hear.

These are only meant to be landmark suggestions based on my experience and those I have known. Your goddess nature ultimately knows best. Listen to it. Just make sure you clear any blind spots to uncovering what's going on and what you need to do to clear it—for all time.

Writing & Journaling

Expressing yourself in written form is a powerful way of connecting to your deepest thoughts and emotions. Many of us find the privacy of a journal or a tablet that is only for our eyes the one place we don't have to censor ourselves. If we're angry, we can write out all the reasons why (and there's sometimes great satisfaction if we decide to burn up or shred those reasons as a way of letting them go). If we're sad, we can express all the reasons, anything from, "No one loves me" to "My spouse no longer makes me happy."

We can write out a sex scene or fantasy as a way of getting in touch with what we want, something I can't recommend highly enough. (You might even consider sharing this with your partner.) You might describe your dream job or dream relationship.

The power of using words consciously can produce miracles. We can heal ourselves. We can illuminate our deepest wishes and desires. We can change how we approach whatever's bothering us. We can manifest something we truly want.

For a long time, I kept a gratitude journal in addition to writing about the various things that bothered me. Every night, I would write down at least three things I was grateful for that had happened that day. I began this practice when I was recovering from a difficult surgery and facing ongoing physical issues. With all of the pain, isolation (I couldn't walk), and physical therapy, it was sometimes a struggle to come up with three items for my journal.

But over the course of my own healing, it became much easier. I got excited when my daily gratitude list grew. Sometimes I could think of as many as ten or twenty things that had happened that day to rock my world. And so my world changed...

The other thing I did in my daily journal was write down all of the things I was doing to better love and heal myself. I even calculated the amount of time I was devoting to it on a daily basis. That changed things too. My life became richer because a part of me needed to see love and growth made tangible. When it was so much a part of me, I didn't need to catalogue it any more. It was just a part of my life. I gave myself what

I needed when I needed it.

Play with what you might need to write or journal about. Maybe it's even writing letters to people that you don't plan on sending. Whatever it is, expressing your thoughts and feelings makes you more present with yourself and your needs. The conversation you have with your goddess woman self will be a beautiful one.

Vision Boards

Just as our written words carry the power of intention, so too do the images with which we surround ourselves. Images can be used to portray something we want, something we believe we will manifest.

You can do a vision board on anything really. I've done ones about my career, my life, my wedding, my home, and even one chronicling pictures of myself at the various stages of my life. I'm an artist to the core, and I love taking an idea I have in my head and finding a picture that represents it.

I used to gather up old magazines from various places and go to town. I cut different sizes and shapes of cardboard, and I would arrange them like a collage. Once I did that, using a combination of words and images, I would place it in a spot in my house that I would see. A specific word or image would catch my eye, giving me a message of what I needed to remember or focus on.

Our higher selves and the Divine are always cheerleading us on, and they will use any available means to communicate with us and get our attention. Let's dive in a little deeper...

Divine Signs & Symbols

The world is as mystical as we allow it to be, and for millennia, people have been paying attention to signs and symbols from the Divine and writing about them. The more I asked for guidance from the Universe, the more things started showing up in *my* universe. I'd see a billboard with a message on it or a catch-phrase in a TV commercial that raised the hairs on my arms.

Then I noticed a white owl on the fence across from my house during the day, something I'd never seen before. Many non-Christian religions have whole books on the symbolic meanings of animals and birds. For example, an owl signifies that you are in touch with your own wisdom—or that you need to be. You get the drift.

Keep an eye out for what's showing up for you. You might be surprised what it tells you or confirms.

Stones & Crystals

What about stones and crystals, you might ask? Really, are we going to go that woo-woo? Yes, because woo-woo is just another story.

I used to think they were just rocks, and that people who liked them were a little woo-woo. Do I love stones and crystals now? You bet.

I discovered their energy accidentally (at least unconsciously). I was in Egypt for business and spent a weekend I had off in Luxor, where I visited an alabaster factory. Two Egyptian men gave me two hunks of that beautiful stone. I was deeply moved, but when I was packing to go home, I thought, "These rocks weigh a ton and what am I going to do with them anyway?"

But I couldn't bring myself to throw them away.

Years later, I was sitting at my computer when I heard one of my guides tell me to pick up the alabaster (yes, I can hear my guides talking to me, although this has been an evolution). For those of you wondering what I'm talking about it, a guide is like your guardian angel or a spirit that's been assigned to help you on your journey, but back to the story...

I went ahead and picked the darn thing up, and wouldn't you know it? For the first time, I could feel energy in what I had thought was an inanimate object.

And it was powerful.

I was also told to look up the meaning of alabaster and discovered it aided in abating anger and encouraging forgiveness, two things I needed help with, especially at that time.

Until then, I didn't know that stones have

energies, and soon I discovered a whole slew of helpers. It blows my mind how much of nature's gifts are related to spiritual support.

My intuition knew what I needed. Yours will too if it's something your goddess nature has planned.

ASTROLOGY

Have you ever looked at your horoscope? Well, astrology has been a guiding force for people for millennia and is chock full of guiding principles and support. If it resonates with you, check it out.

I kinda didn't know what I was getting into when a healer suggested I contact her friend to have my birth chart read, but when I heeded her advice, my mind was blown. She'd given me a map of who I was as a goddess woman and the lessons my soul had arranged for me in this life. I was moved to tears when I finished listening.

The accuracy was mind-blowing, and all she'd had to go on was my birth date and time of my birth.

I like to think that the Divine arranged for us each to have our own private life map in the stars at the moment of our birth. Certainly in centuries past, this birth map was considered to be a powerful source of wisdom to guide one's life.

Yoga & Other Physical Practices

Yoga has become one of the most popular practices to connect the body with the spirit. The movements are designed to open up the body's energies, but other practices like Qi gong and tai chi do so as well.

Like everything else, when you add love and intention to anything, you take it to a higher level. I have always found that to be the case with these practices.

Energy Healing & Other Modalities

How about alternate energy modalities? I have found acupuncture to be wonderful, but once I discovered energy healing, it was like a super-charged rocket had blazed through my life.

I shifted easier and faster from old beliefs and cleared blockages in ways that served my highest good. I got down to the root causes instead of band-aiding issues or moving or clearing energy that showed up time and time again.

When my own healing gifts blew into my life, I found myself helping others in the same way. If you need it, I can't recommend it enough. Your goddess nature will lead you to the right people. I also note a few healers I have personally worked with on my website.

Trust Your Intuition

Looking for more tips? Pay attention to where your hand unconsciously rests on your body, or what your intuition is telling you to do.

Your goddess nature will always show you the way.

Enjoy the ride, goddess woman.

It truly is a wonderful life.

THE GODDESS GUIDES
TO BEING A WOMAN

Read the whole collection...

Goddesses Decide:
Relearning Divine Power

Stop buying all the lies that say you can't have the life you want. You're a goddess woman. Reclaim your true power.

Goddesses Deserve The Gs:
Linking Self-Worth with Material Abundance

Become the goddess moneymaker you were born to be. Believe you're worth all the abundance you set your sights on.

Goddesses Love Cock:
Re-establishing the Divine Connection

Get it on like a goddess! Bring joy and connection back into the bedroom.

Goddesses Cry and Say Motherfucker:
Erasing Shame from Human Expression

Forget all you've learned about getting angry or sad and everything in between... Express yourself like a goddess.

Goddesses Don't Do Drama:
Removing Toxicity from Relationships

Say no to toxic peeps and all their crap and start building the loving and joyful relationships you truly want.

Goddesses Are Sexy:
Enjoying a Loving Self-Image

Delete all the stories saying you aren't beautiful or sexy. Start believing it today!

Goddesses Eat:
Reclaiming a Divine Partnership with Food

Throw off all the soul-sucking stories about food. Learn to feast like a goddess woman.

Goddesses Are Happy:
Living a Fulfilling Life
Find your inner happy place as a goddess woman. Start enjoying life!

Goddesses Face Fear:
Tapping into Divine Courage
Face down your fears and demons like a goddess woman. Tap into your innate courage!

MORE GODDESS GUIDES ARE COMING...

Sign up for my newsletter www.avamiles.com to keep up-to-date for your next powerful goddess woman shift.

GODDESS MEMO FROM AVA

HEY GODDESS WOMAN!

Thank you for sharing The Goddess Guides journey with me! It's a joy to be connected to a divine rockstar like you.

If you leave a review, I want to thank you up front. Every time a reader takes the time out of her busy schedule to share her feelings about my books, I'm so grateful.

And if you decide to tell friends or co-workers about The Goddess Guides because they just have to read them... Well, you've changed your world and helped more women become the goddess women they want to be. From one goddess woman to another, I want to bless you for it. And you will be. Trust me.

Until we meet again, have fun being your amazing goddess woman self.

Lots of love,

Ava

AUTHOR BIO

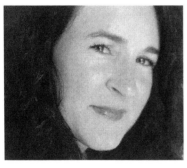 International bestselling author Ava Miles calls herself a divine rockstar—something she believes everyone is deep down. Ava spent many years traveling the world and sharing her gifts with women and men in war-torn countries, helping them to rebuild and reintegrate their communities amidst intense struggle. She has managed multi-million-dollar projects for international agencies, such as the United Nations.

Now, she brings that experience together with her passion for sparking joy and personal success in people's lives in *The Goddess Guides to Being A Woman*.

For more information about Ava, visit www.avamiles.com.

47118981R00125

Made in the USA
Middletown, DE
16 August 2017